LEARNING TOGETHER

Healthy NUTRITION AND LIFE SKILLS

Step by Step...

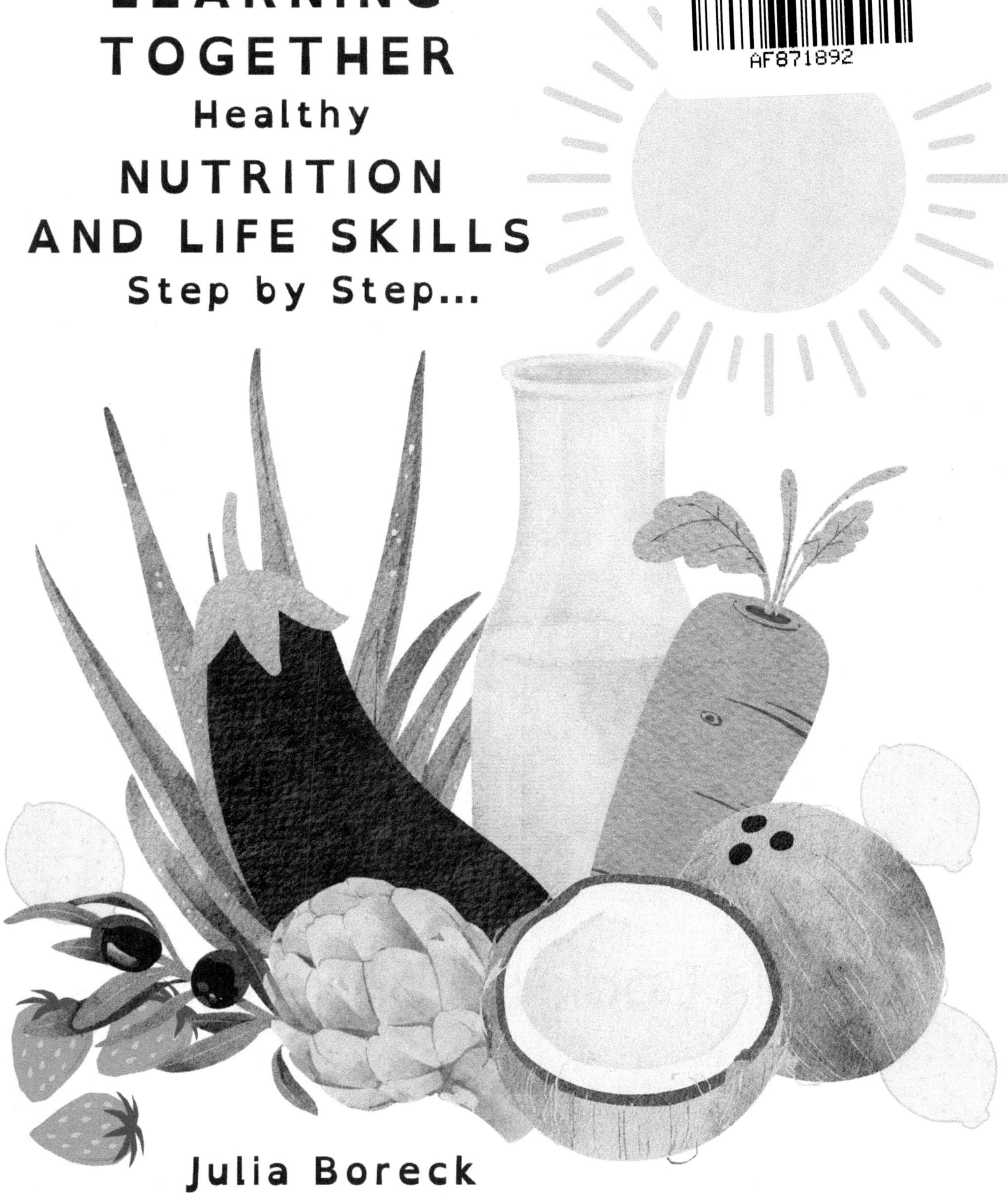

Julia Boreck

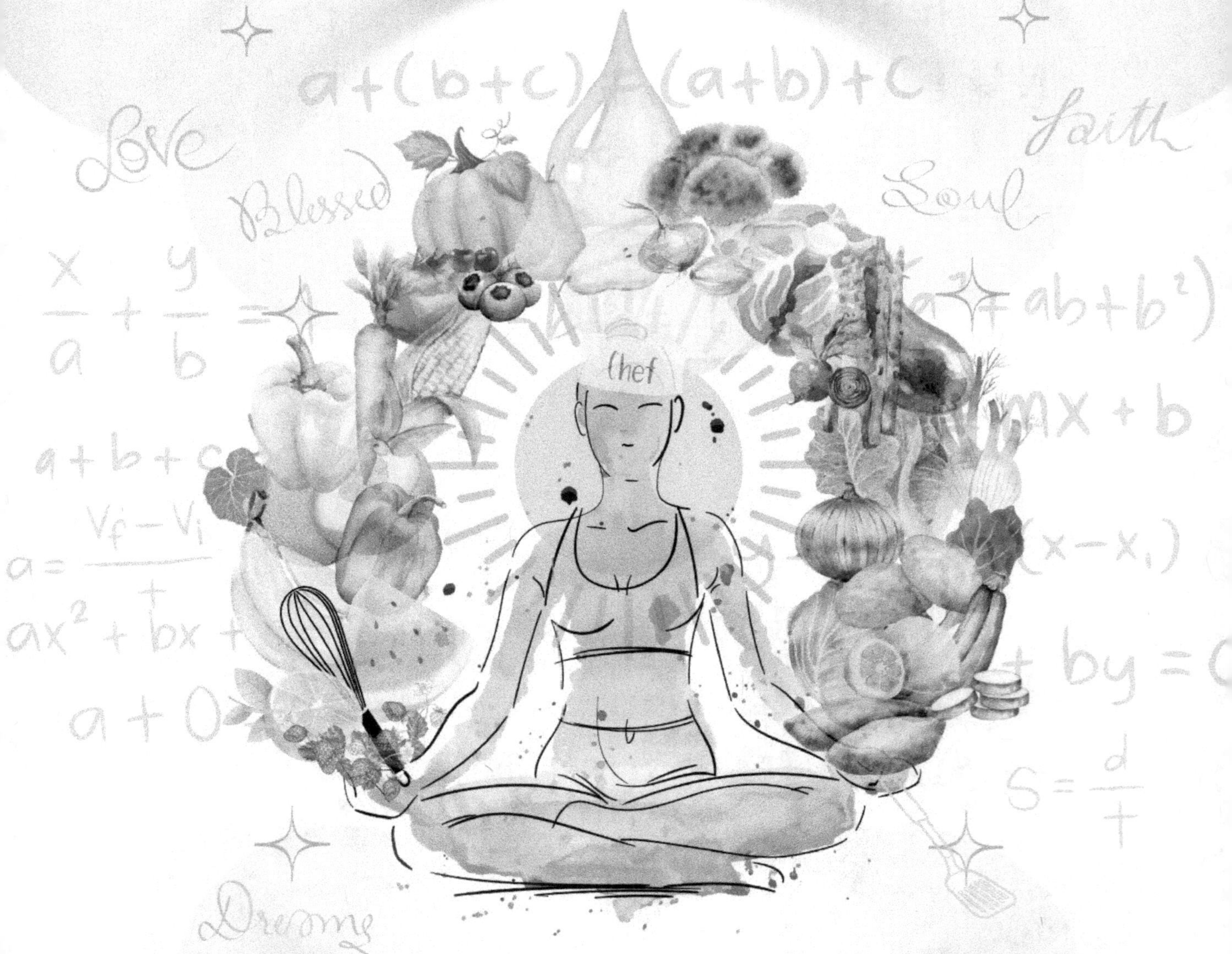

This Book Belongs to:

____

ABOUT ME

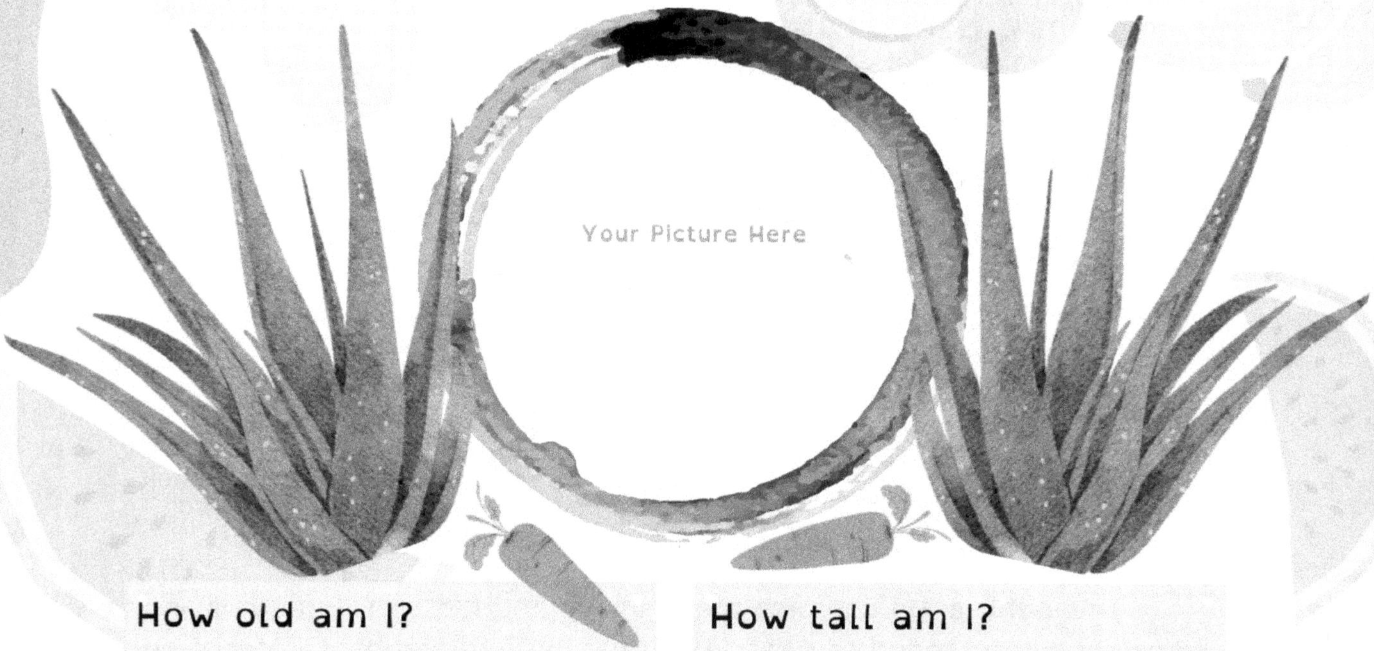

How old am I?

How tall am I?

Favorites Foods:

Favorite Activities:

Favorite Quote:

A fun fact about me is:

This book is dedicated to my daughter,
the one who teaches and reminds
me daily the simplicity and
beauty of love.

I love you!

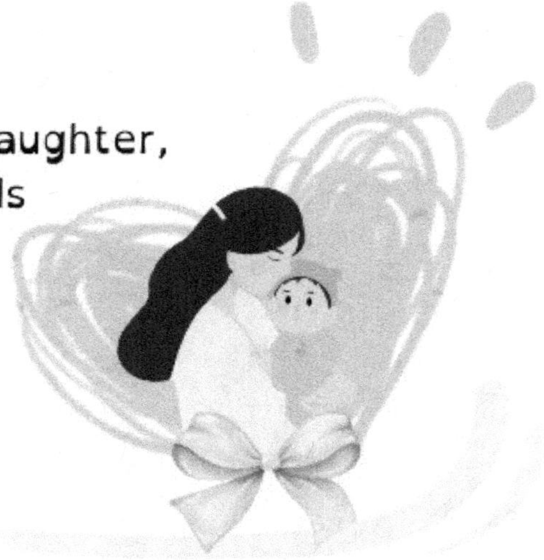

Updated 2026
ISBN 9798988622581

This publication contains the opinions and ideas of its author and research. It is intended to provide helpful and informational material on the subjects addressed in the publication. It is sold with the understanding that the author and publisher are not engaged in rendering medical, health, financial, or any other kind of personal professional services in this book. Any statements or claims about the possible health benefits in this book have not been evaluated by the Food and Drug Administration and are not intended to diagnose, treat, cure or prevent disease.

Information in this book is meant to motivate reader to make healthy choices based on the reader's own research in partnership with his or her healthcare provider. It should not be relied upon to determine dietary changes, a medical diagnosis, or courses of treatment. The content of this book is not intended to be a substitute for professional medical advice, diagnosis, or treatment. Always seek the advice of your nutritionist, doctor, or other qualified health care provider with any questions you have regarding a medical condition. Never disregard professional medical advice or delay in seeking it because of something you have read in this book. Reliance on information provided by this book or elsewhere is solely at your own risk.

The author and publisher specifically disclaim all responsibility for any liability, loss, or risk, personal or otherwise, that is incurred as a consequence. Directly or indirectly, of the use and application of any of the contents of this book.

What You Will Achieve

Through the pages of this book,
you will gain confidence in yourself, have knowledge to wisely choose foods that will nourish your body, mind, energy, and mood, and begin to think creatively on making positive changes for yourself and in the lives around you.
Fueling yourself with proper energy through food, thought, and action lead to creating a more joyful, confident, and balanced life.
Keeping yourself healthy is a way of loving and nourishing yourself inside and out.
Have fun exploring and learning these pages and beyond. Remember, you are a bright, beautiful, and intelligent being that has the ability to learn, grow, excel in life, and inspire those around you!

Dream Big Live Big

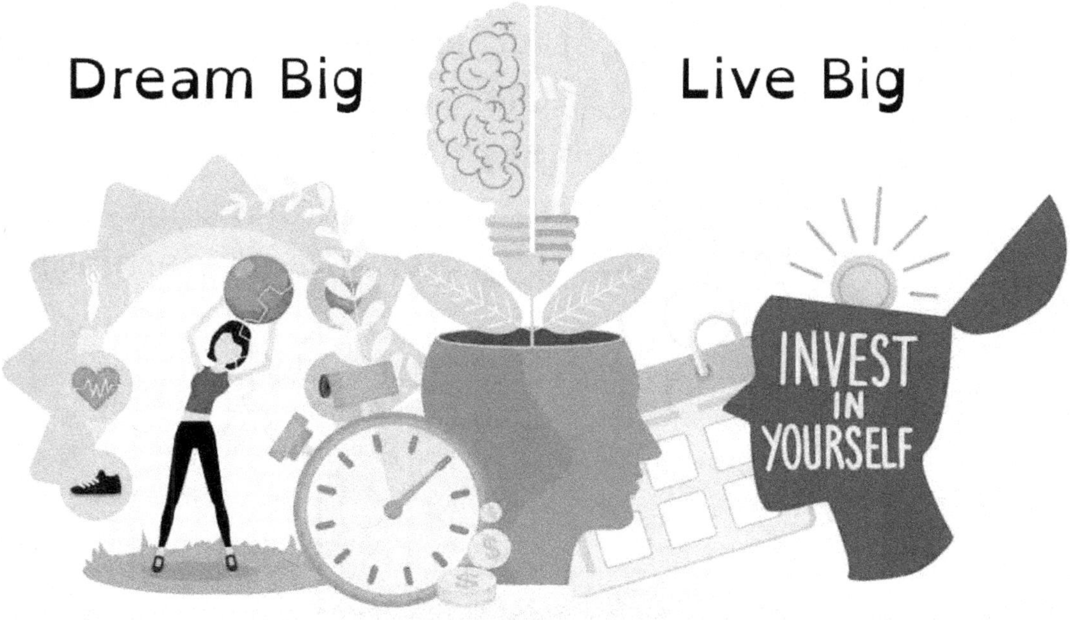

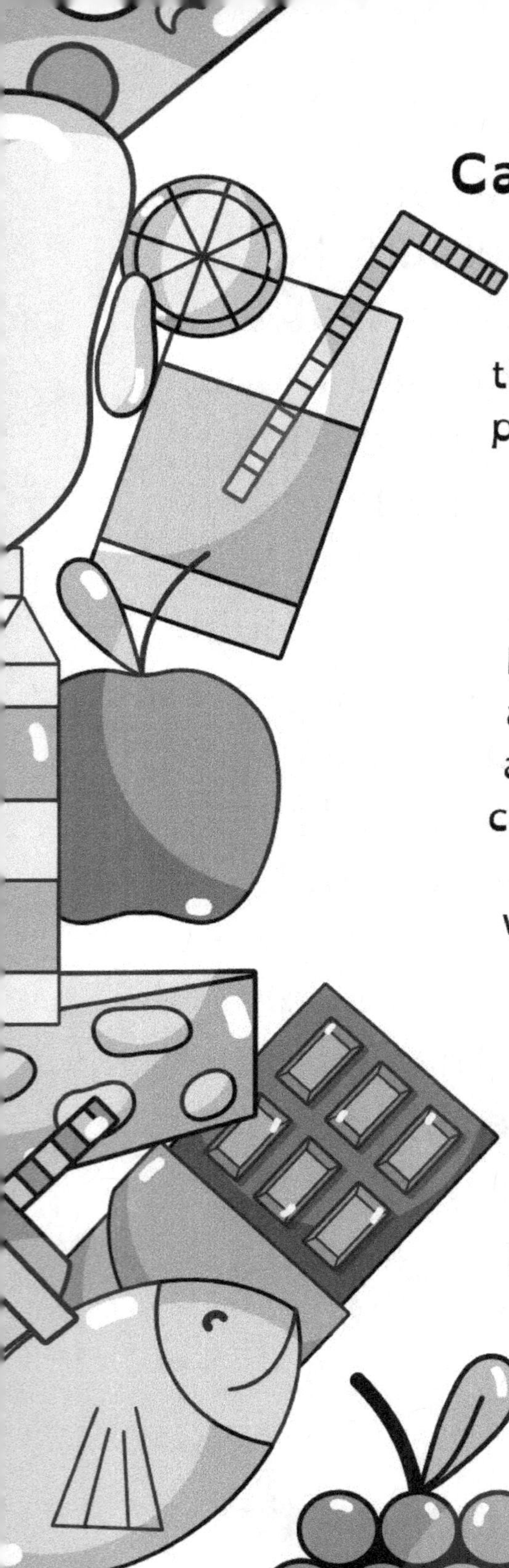

A Note on Research, Caregivers, Guidance, & Help

As you research the answers to questions, use your resources from the web, encyclopedias, history books, people, and so forth... having a variety of resources is great! Remember to site your resources as a way to go back and trace your steps.

In the kitchen, think responsibly, seek assistance when needed, be informed about food safety, like avoiding cross contamination. When you are unsure of something, listen to your intuition, wait, research, and ask for help. This is all part of the learning journey.

When questions come up across the math, reading, writing prompts, and other subjects, be sure to give your best answers, then check for help, correction, and other feedback. In life, there are no answer keys, so just keep trying, ask questions, be okay with a little uncertainty, keep going, growing, and learning!

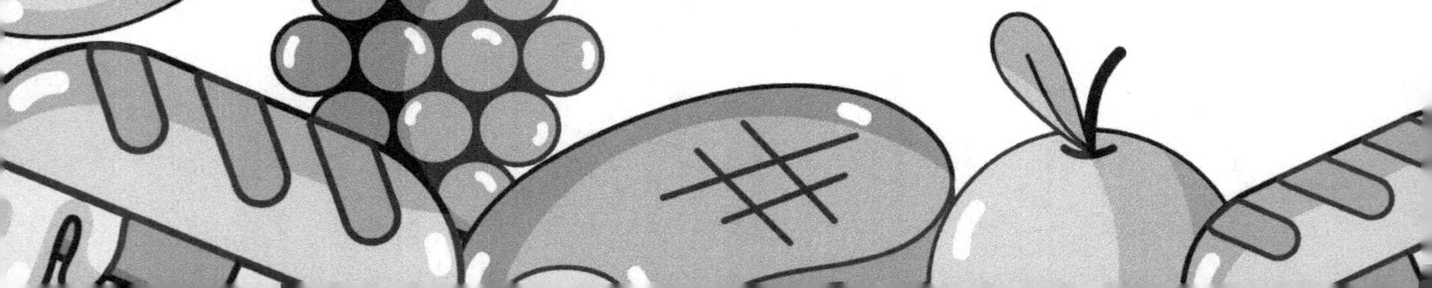

TABLE OF CONTENTS

What is Health?	9
Health Evaluation	12
Mood & Food	15
Food Pyramid	17
Let Your Garden Grow	20
Herb Garden	25
Power of Tea	27
Breathing Techniques	28
Affirmations	29
All About Produce	30
Edible Parts of Plants	31
Fruit or Vegetable	35
Produce Color Wheel	40
Brain Smoothie	41
Fruit Math	44
Still Life Drawings	46
Cleaning Produce	49
Fifteen Clean	55
A Dozen Dirty	59
Why Organic?	67
Pollination	72
The Flower's Journey	77
Cucumber Pucker	80
Food Measurements	82
Reduse, Reuse, Recycle	84
The Recycle King	87
Backyard Chickens	90
Appeal in Peels	91
Sweet Green Smoothie	93
Pineapple Business	96
Pineapple Math	98
Running with Numbers	100
Planning	102
Tropical Smoothie	104
Got Grain on the Brain	107
Grain Search	108
Grainy Breakdown	111
Making Bread	115
Grainy Math	123
The Flour Journey	126
Nutrition On The Go	130
Granola Fun Recipe	133
Fun Foods	135
Mindful Eating	139
Kitchen Conversions	141
Superfood Heroes	146
Chia Pudding Recipe	153
Supercado Spa	157
Cacao Smoothie	160
Antioxidant Alley	163

TABLE OF CONTENTS

Vitamin Valley	166
Alley, Valley, & Mine	169
Got Dairy	173
Nut Milk Recipe	179
Say Cheese	181
Butter on the Move	185
Butter Cream Math	188
Yogurt	189
Power of Gut Health	192
Berry Good Parfait	196
Alkaline Abbey	199
Alkaline Foods	202
PRAL Tool	205
Acid or Alkaline?	208
Balanced Lifestyle	209
Alkaline Lemon Icey	213
Protein	216
Amino Acids	220
Serving Protein	222
Beans & Legumes	226
Nutty Benefits	231
Nutty Ideas	232
Nutty Trivia	233
Nutty Smoothie Recipe	235
Underwater Food	238
Gone Fishing	240
Land Food	242
Chicken	245
Pork	246
Beef	247
Protein Math	248
Protein Meal Plan	252
Got Muscle?	255
Meal Plan for You!	256
Drink Up	259
Water Science	262
Types of Wet Water	268
Healthy Juice	270
Melon Slush Recipe	272
Popsicle Freeze	275
The Finale	279
Reflect & Goal Setting	280
Your Nutritional Chart	281
Food Truck Business	284
Design Time	285
Food Truck Event	291
Dream Stage Principles	295
Time To Celebrate	299

What Is Health?

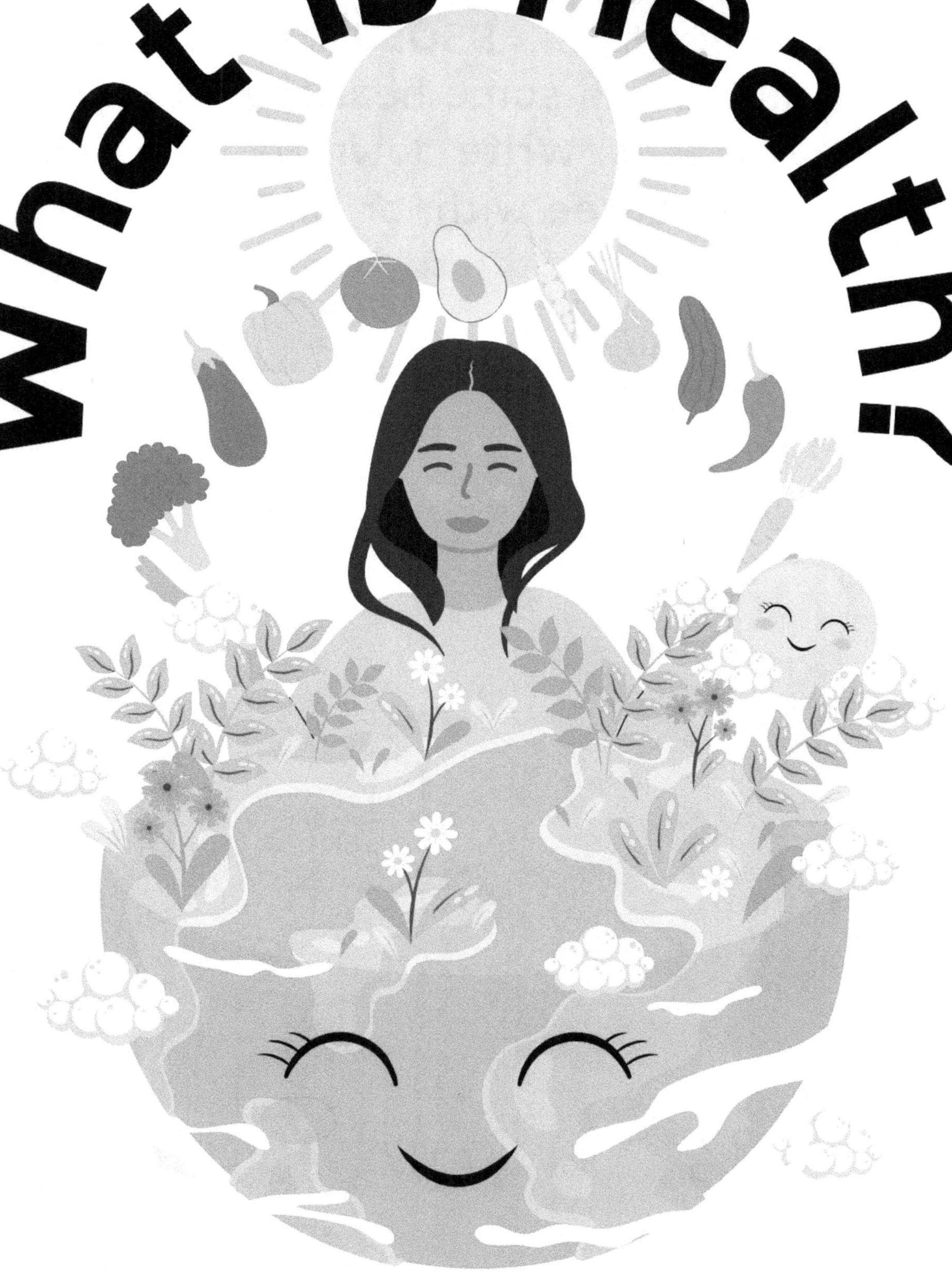

Health is many things added up that compose of your overall wellbeing. Your health is ABSOLUTELY important!

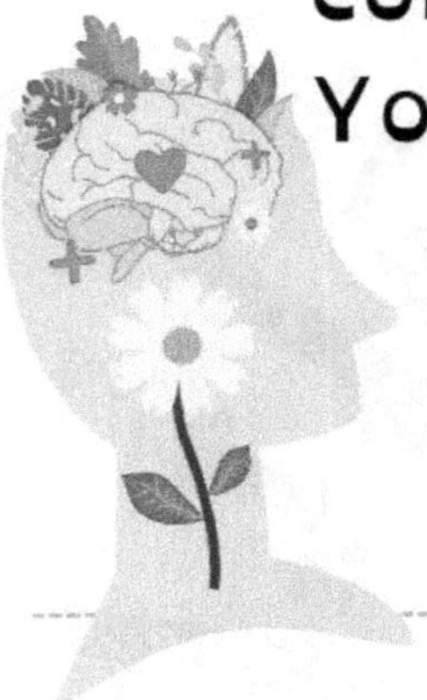

Research some health quotes and phrases. Write down the ones you like, agree with, or find inspiring.

Health is your wealth, spend wisely.

Who is Dr. Sebi?

What does Dr. Sebi have to say?

What does health mean to you?

Research and write what health means and how to maintain a healthy diet and lifestyle.

Practice your cursive handwriting skills!

Got Health?

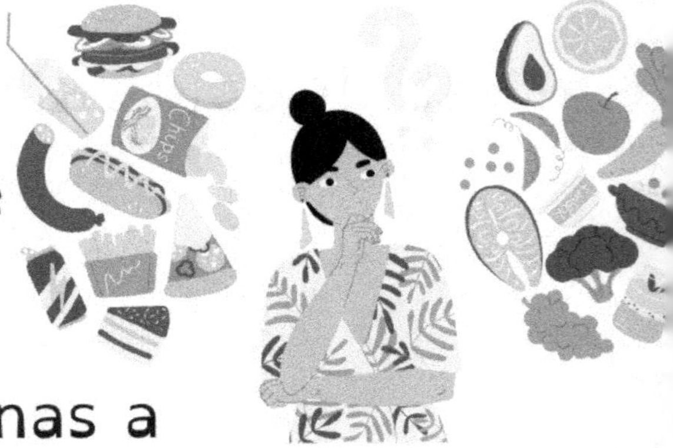

How often do you eat these foods? Next to each item write how often you eat them. If you eat three bananas a week, write "3 x week" next to the bananas.

Got Health?

How often do you practice these healthy habits? Next to each item write how often you do them. For example, if you swim two times a week, write "2 x week" next to the picture.

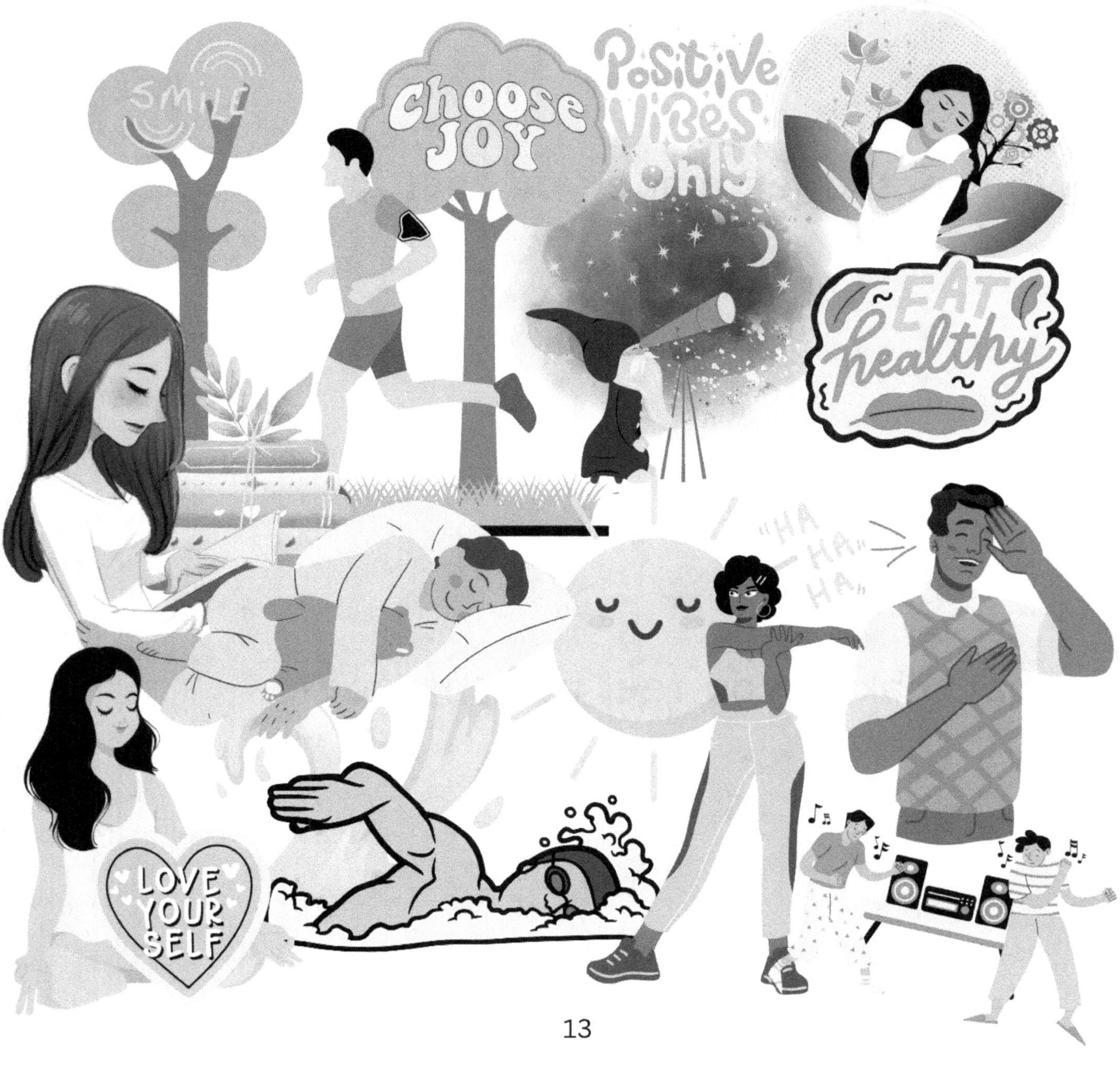

What foods make you feel great?

What activities make you feel great?

What makes you feel not so good?

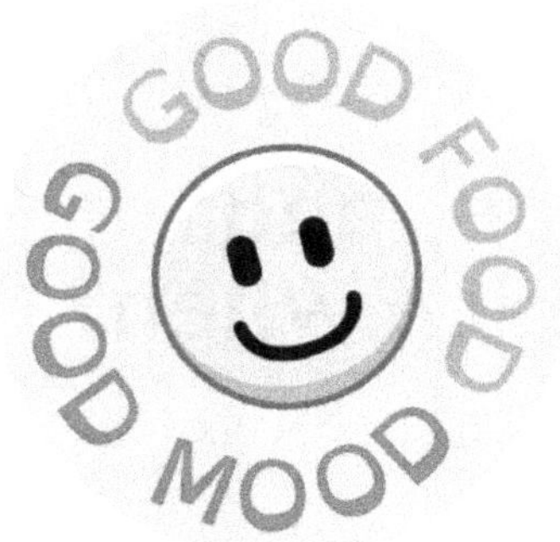

In several studies revolving around people eating "junk food" there is a strong connection between eating unhealthy foods and negative effects of both mind and body, including weight gain and depression. Interestingly enough, the opposite is true for healthy foods. Have you experienced or seen this? Explain.

Research and explain what the SAD diet is. Is this healthy? Do you eat like this?

Research, "Let food be thy medicine, and medicine be thy food." Who wrote it? When? What does it mean?

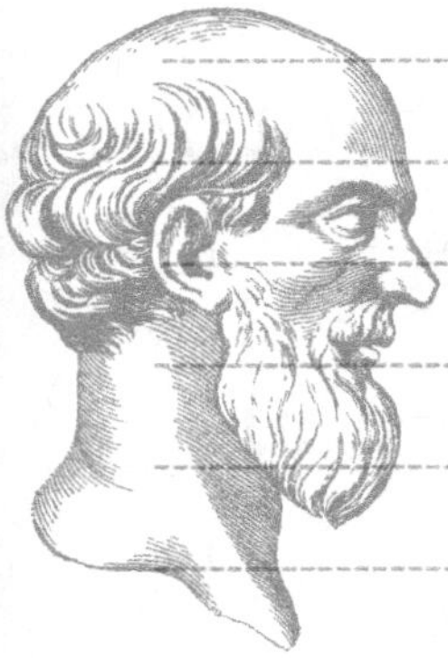

What was Leonardo da Vinci's concept of health. Write down what you find.

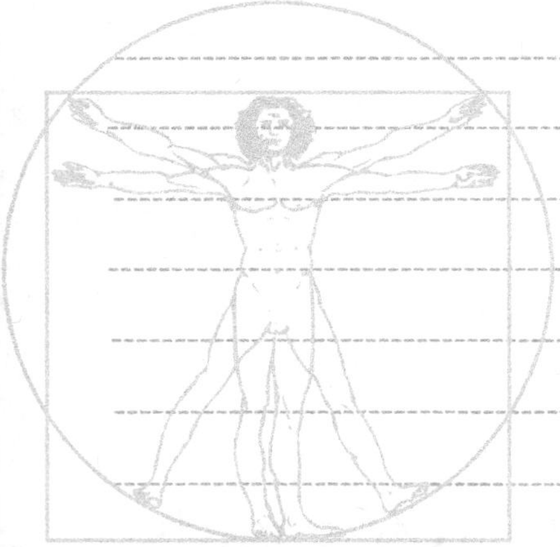

How important are food, mood, and good habits toward keeping healthy?

Food Pyramid

Research and fill in the food pyramid.

Which categories did you include?

Did you include exercise? Explain.

Did you include fluids? Explain.

Did you include rest? Explain.

Did you include mood? Explain.

Research a ‘food pyramid’ from another country. Describe the similarities and differences from the one you had researched previously. Do you agree with one more than the other?

How would you make a completely different 'food pyramid'? Example, a health chart with half food and half healthy activities.

Let Your Garden Grow

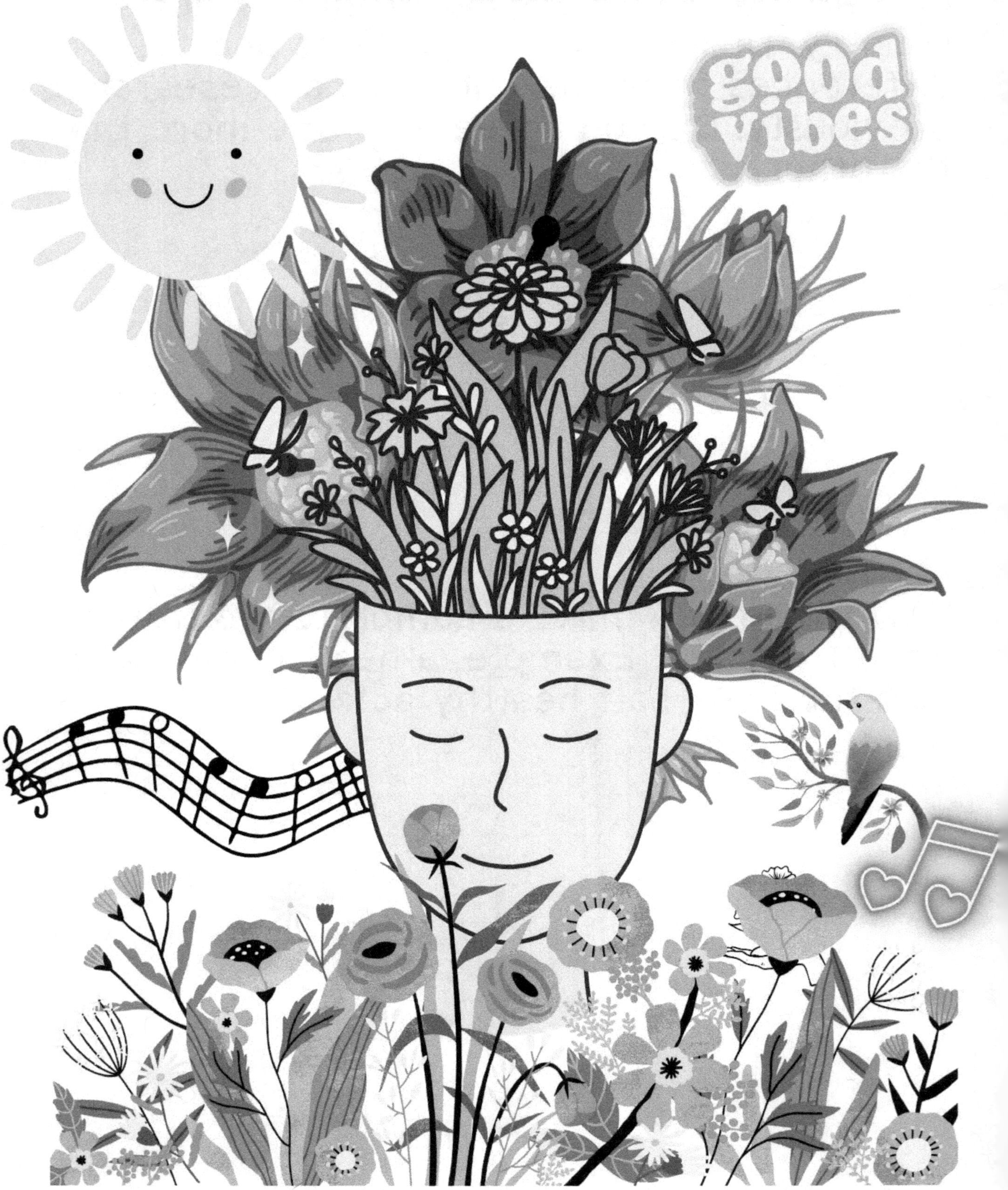

Getting your hands and feet in Mother Earth's soil and absorbing the beautiful warm sun rays from above can be a very rich, fulfilling, calming, and nourishing activity especially when you reap the benefits of your harvest! We can get a great dose of vitamin D from the sun, why is this vitamin so important?

Explain how vitamin D is linked to mood and well-being.

Explain how stepping outside barefoot also can be very healthy for the mind, body, and soul.

Can gardening be seen as a form of healthy exercise? Explain the research.

Outdoors, in nature, under the sun, gardening, exercising...What else do you need to have a great time?
Shaded area...Birds singing...Picnic...
Breezes blowing...Music...

Does music effect people's mood, self-esteem, and energy? Explain.

Can music play a role in the growth of plants? Research and describe.

Do you think people and plants respond to positive words and affirmations?

Based on your gardening climate zone, what edible plants could you grow in your area?

Name a few edible plants you can grow inside your home.

What kind of music would you play your plants?

What positive affirmations would you say or have written around the plants?

Thyme to play some music for your indoor **herb garden.** Match the herb name with the picture. Now pick a few to grow!

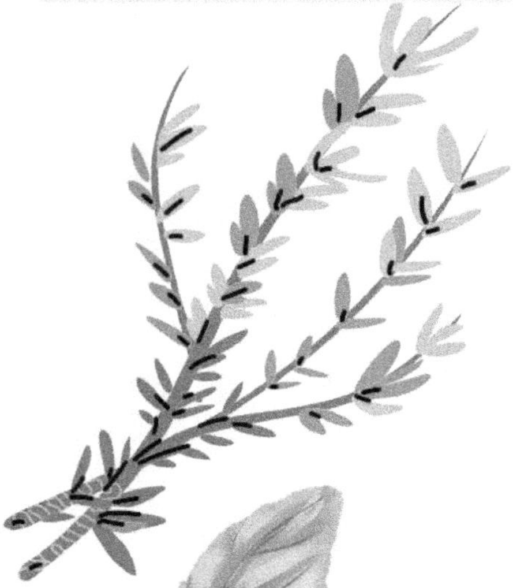

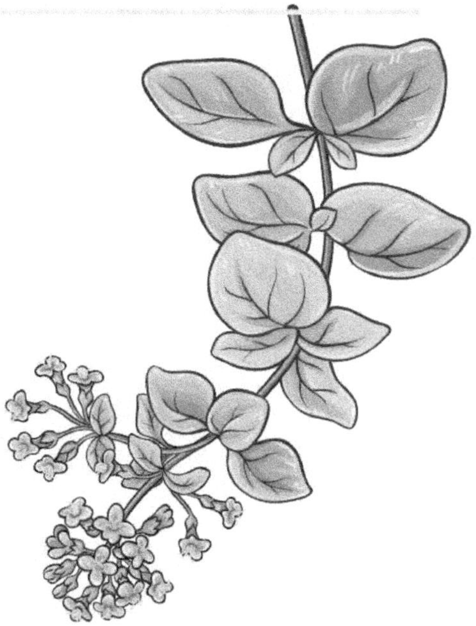

Mint

Chives

Parsley

Oregano

Basil

Sage

Rosemary

Thyme

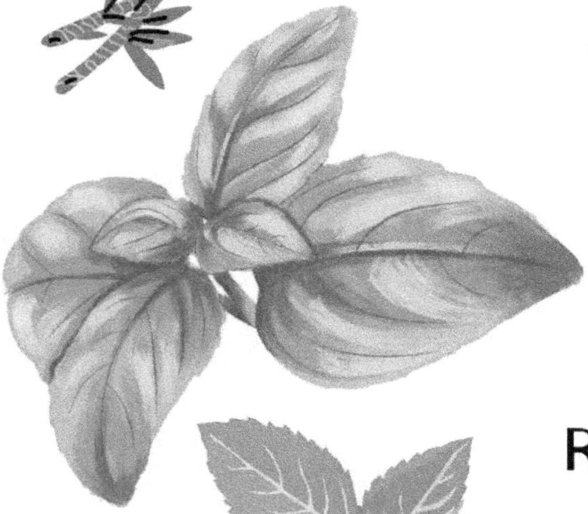

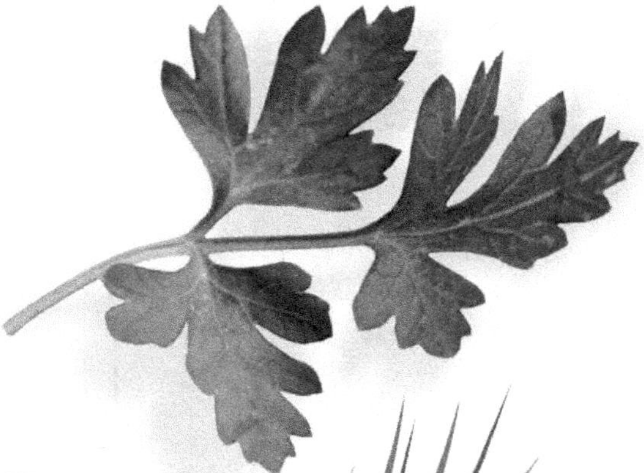

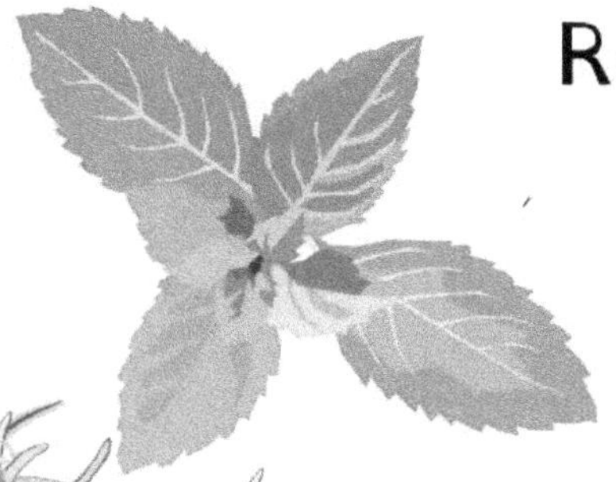

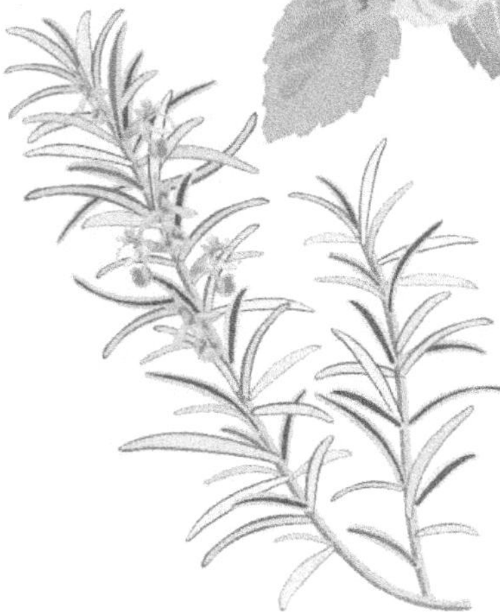

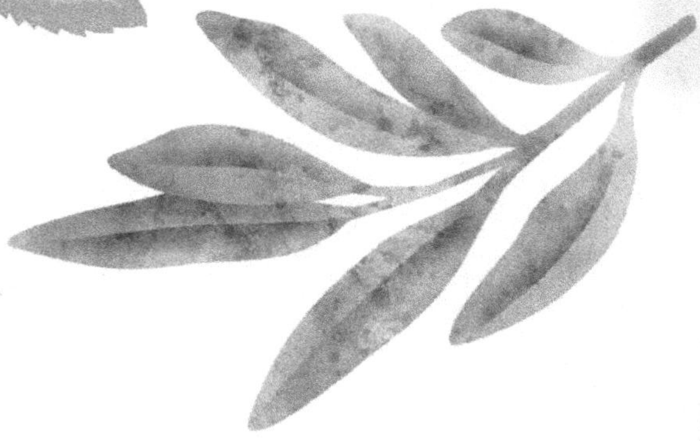

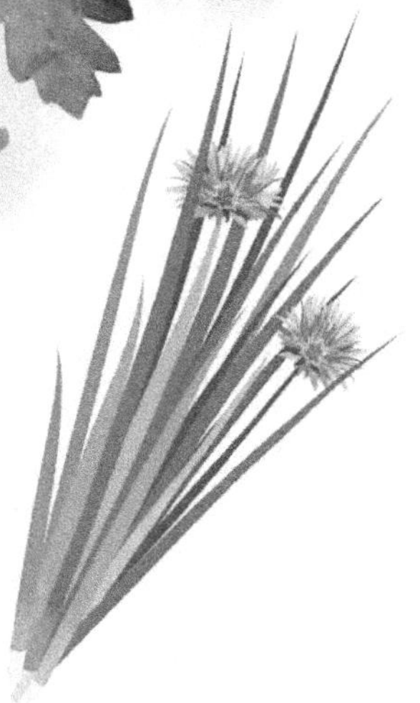

Research and write the nutritional or medicinal benefits of these herbs.

CHAMOMILE

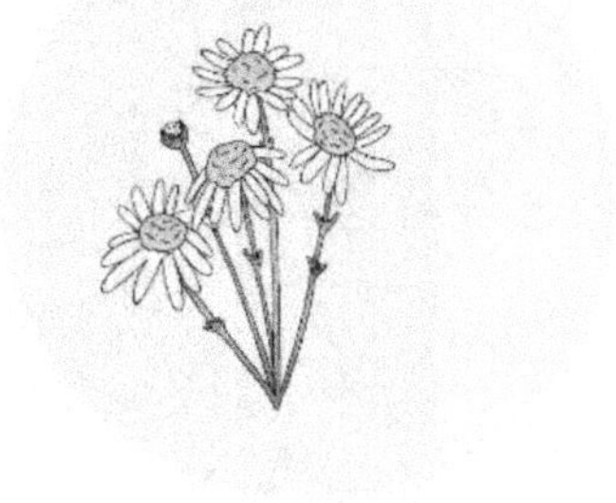

LEMONGRASS

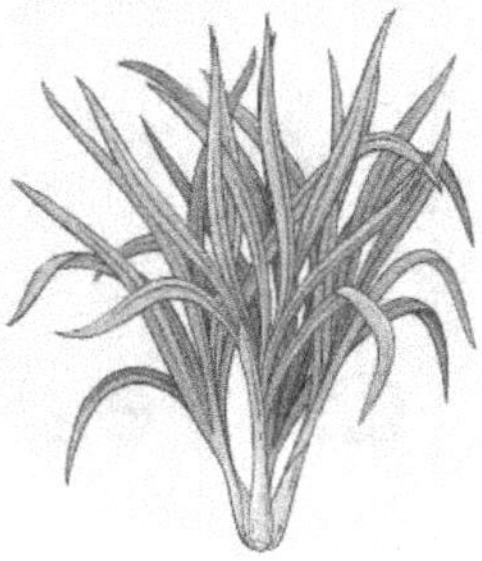

CHIVES

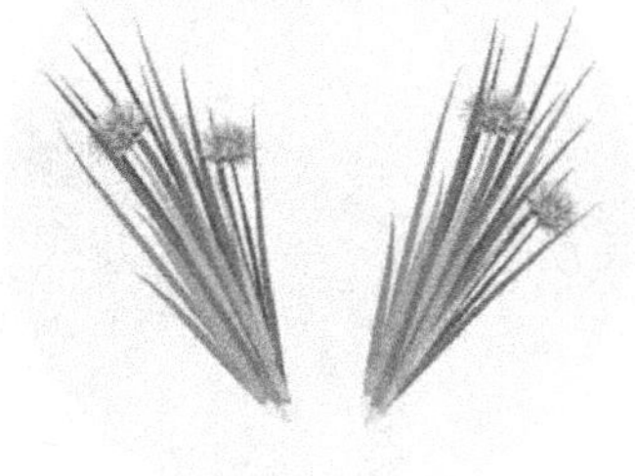

ROSEMARY

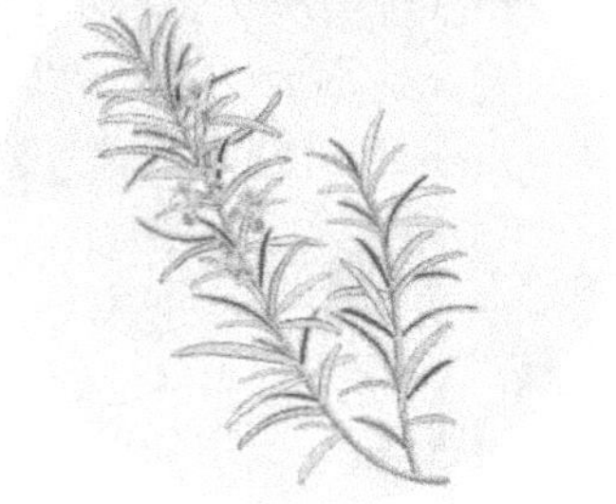

LAVENDER

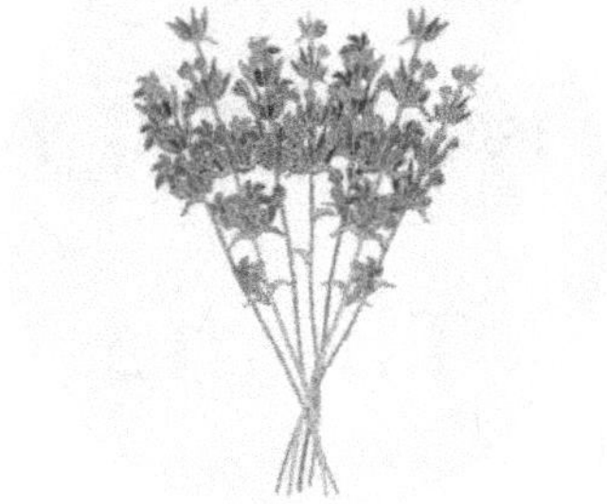

CILANTRO

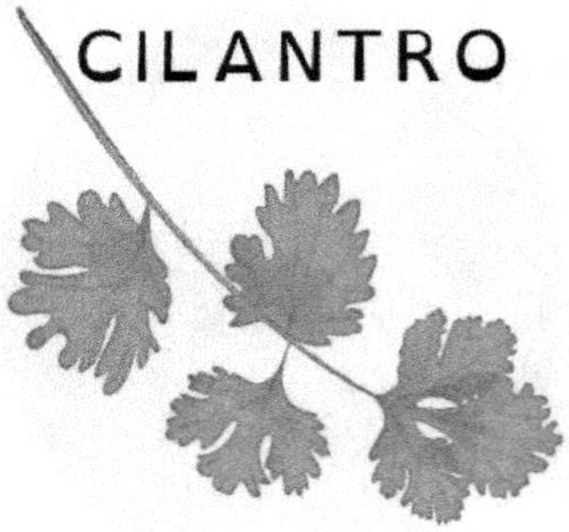

Breathe and Sip into the Zone

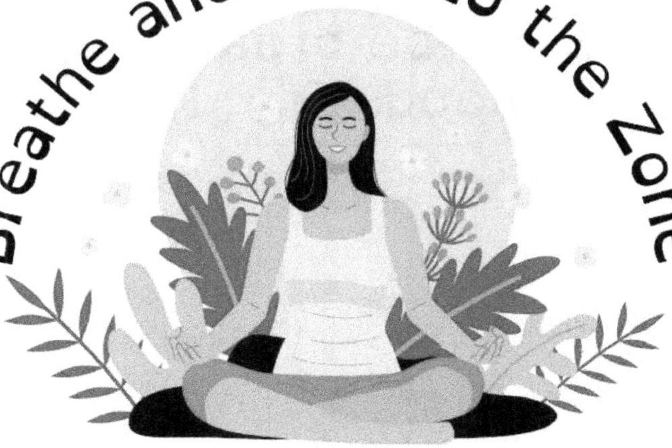

Tea can be an amazing way to unwind or even wind up. Next to each mood or situation, find an herbal tea ingredient that is used as a medicinal aid. Take a sip, how do you feel?

Calm		
Sleep Aid		
Energy Boost		
Happy		
Rid Anxiety		
Boost Immunity		
Stomach Ache		
Increase Focus		
Muscle & Joint		

Research and describe **breathing techniques** to achieve each mood. Try, how do you feel?

Tranquility

Increase Focus

Energy Boost

Love Breath

Try this calming breathing whistle, tuned at the frequency of love (528 Hz). With each exhale you hear it's sound! Practice releasing tension and gaining clarity with this breath work necklace that comes with a free self-care journal download.

Knowing yourself and how to effectively face situations as they arrive takes time, practice, repetition, and staying positive in your mindset, the words you choose, and the actions you take will all help build the skills for success. It may take many times for something to make sense or flow smoothly. Just stay on track. Write a few **affirmations** that help when you face challenging times.

I believe in myself.
I can do this.
I have the power to change and grow.

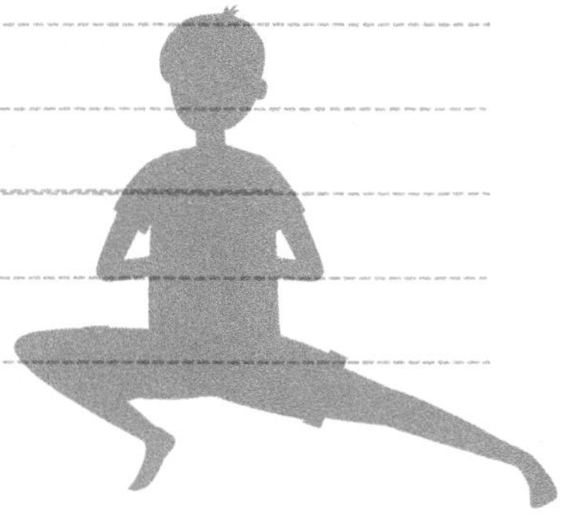

All About Produce

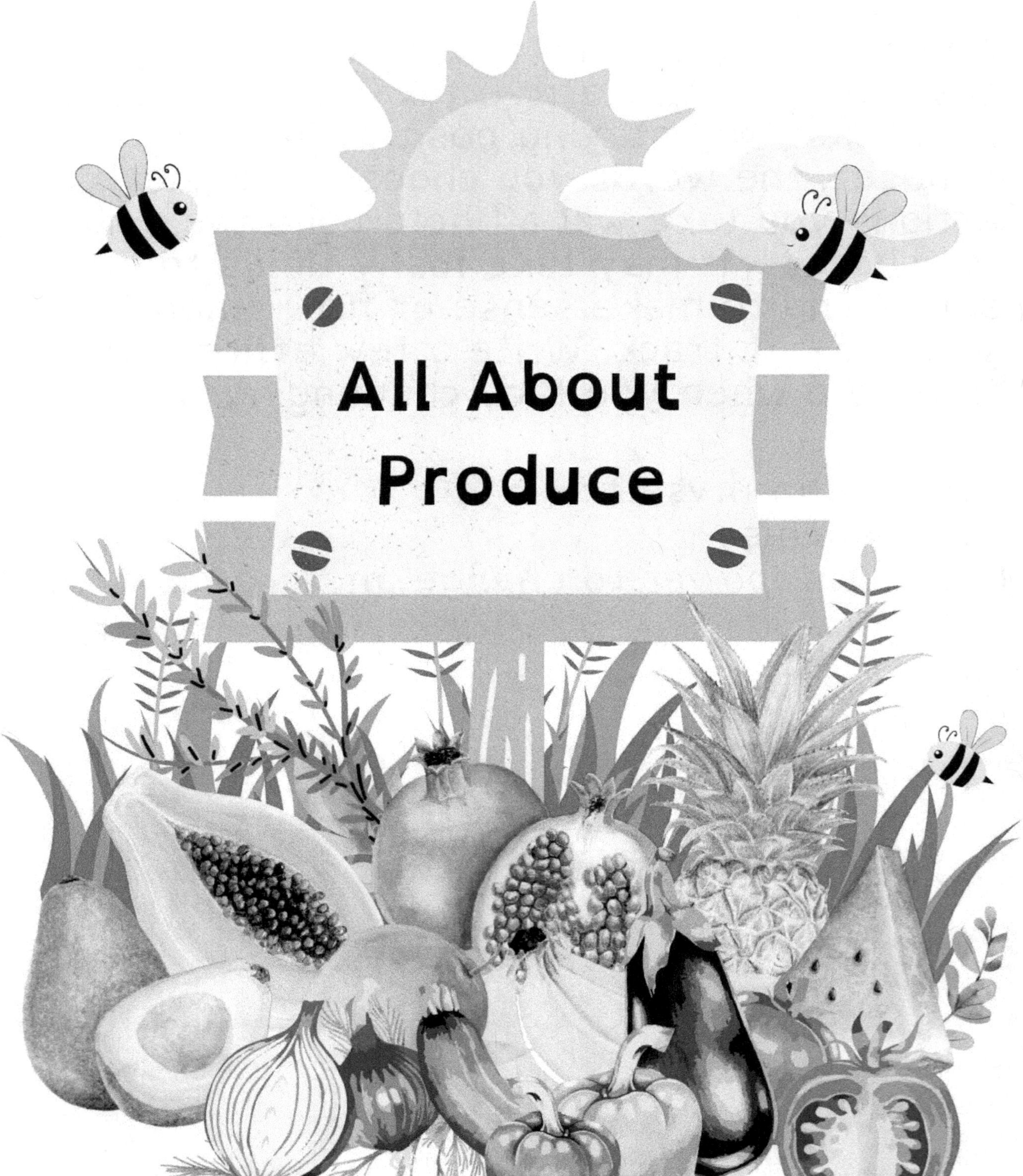

Edible Parts of Plants

People eat many parts of plants. Identify which part of the plant the following foods come from, using these terms:

STEM

SEED

FRUIT

ROOTS

LEAVES

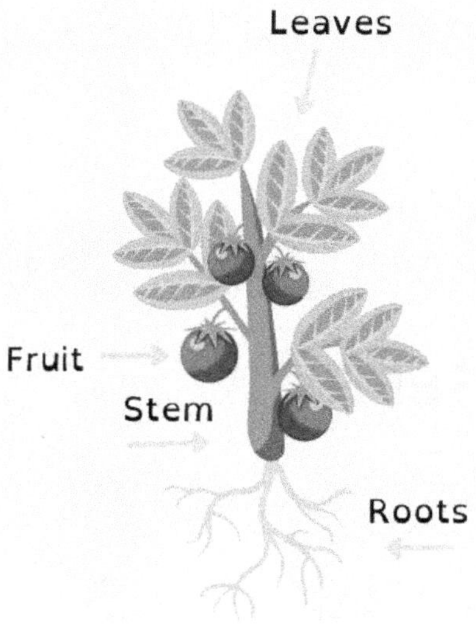

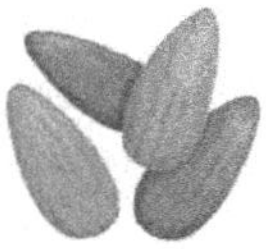

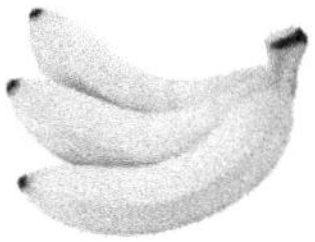

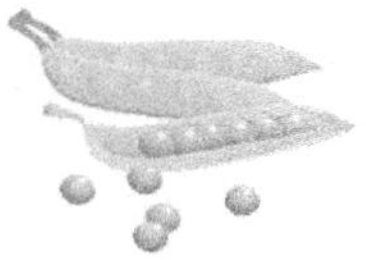

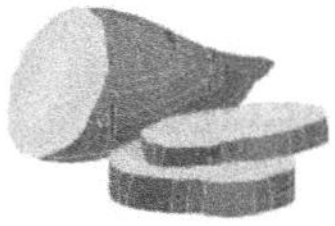

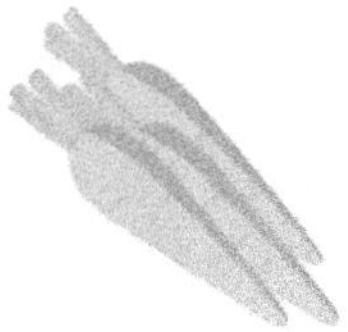

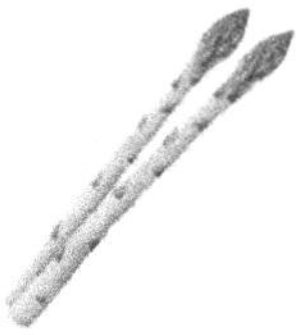

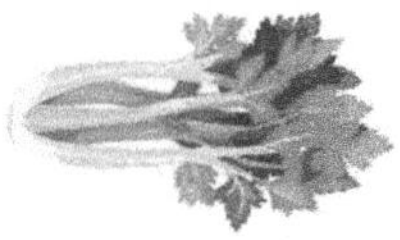

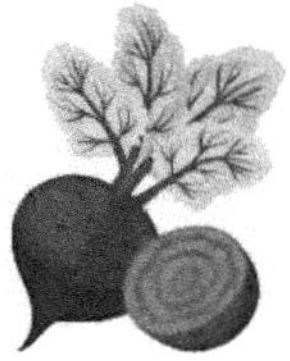

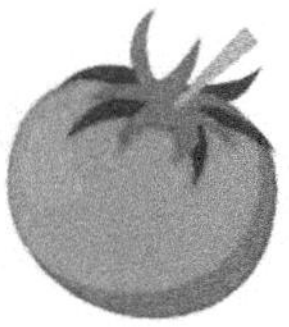

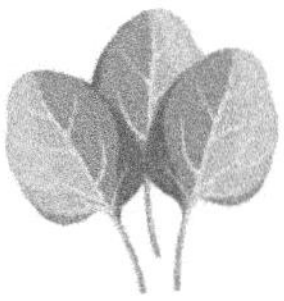

Research and write foods in each category.

STEM:

SEED:

FRUIT:

ROOT:

LEAF:

What Is This?

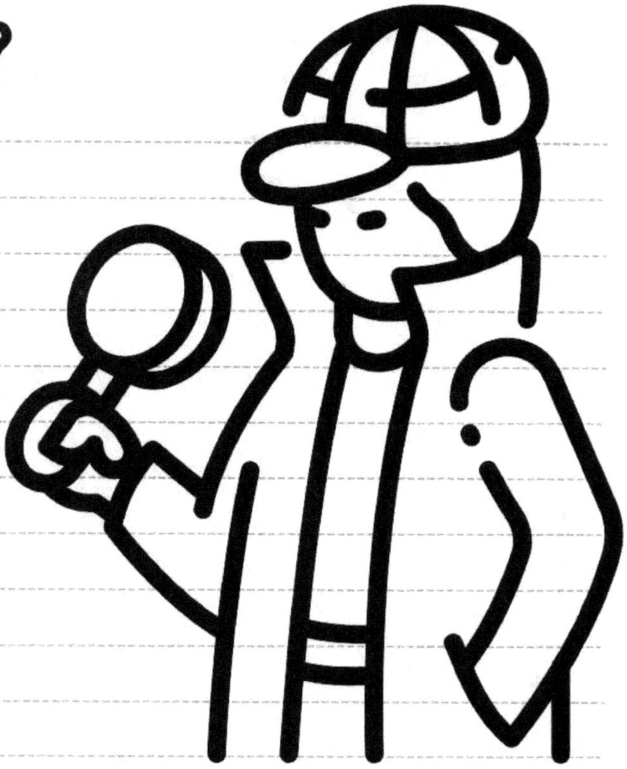

I can be put into teas.

I am a root.

I have anti-inflammatory properties.

I am not spicy.

If I have curcumin, what am I?

What medicinal properties do I have? (In other words, how can I help people?)

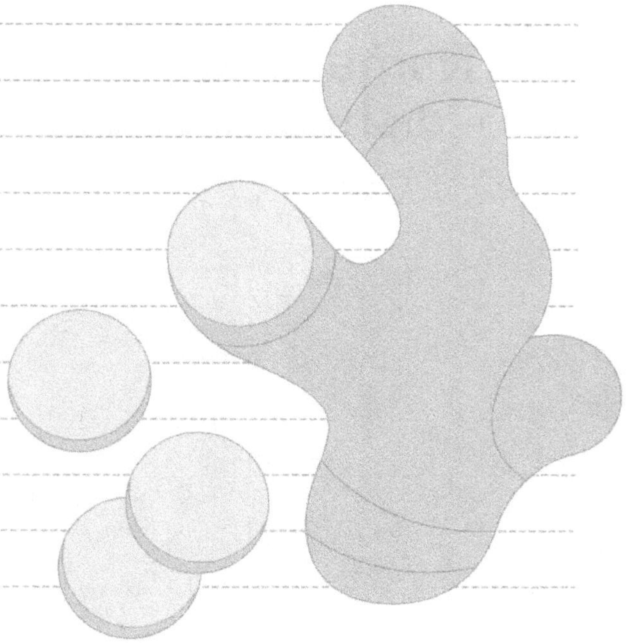

Similar, But Different

Write about ginger and turmeric.

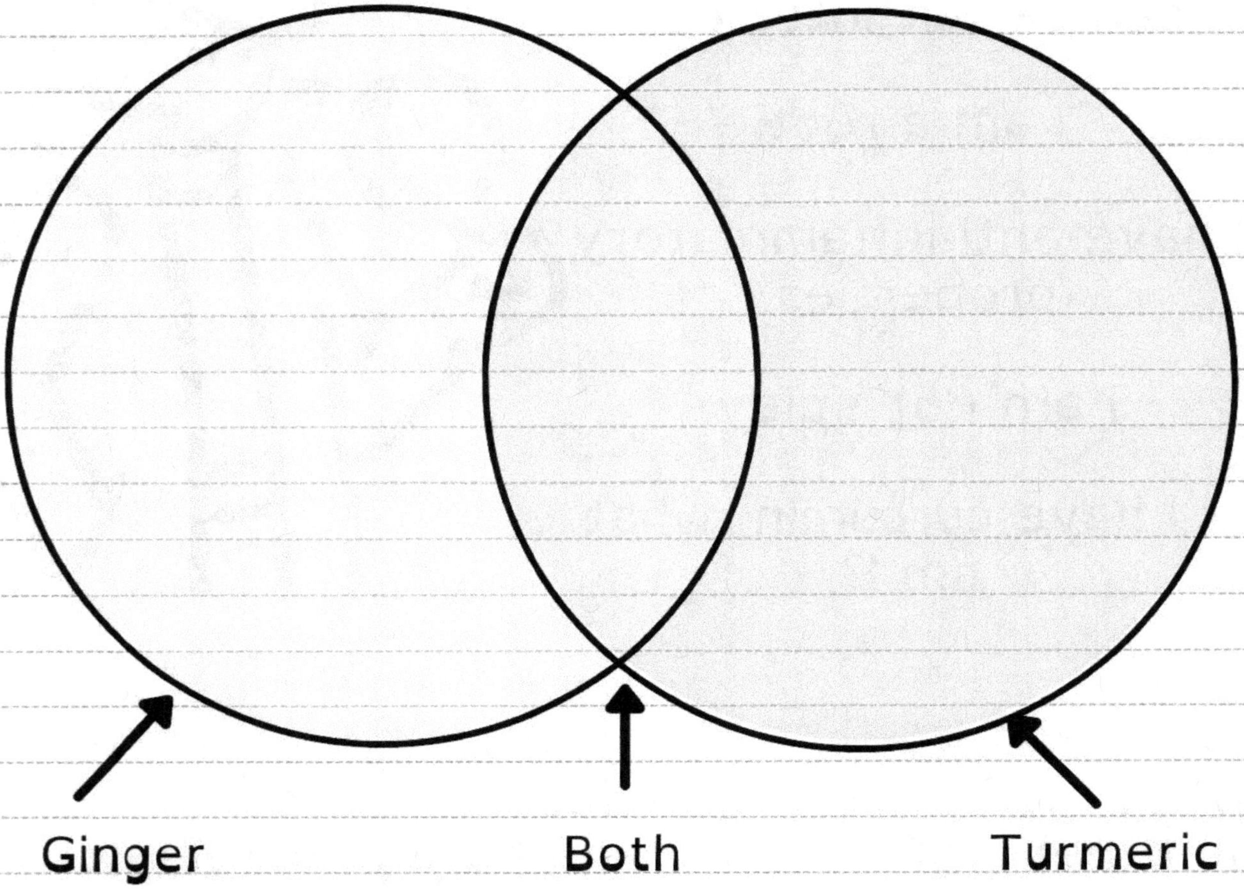

Name a few sweet and savory foods and dishes that use these nutritious roots.

Fruit or Vegetable?

Color the vegetables green and the fruits red. Be careful, these are tricky!

Cicle the word if it is a fruit and underline the word if it is a vegetable. Put these on your Fruit & Vegetable Color Wheel on page 40.

Golden Kiwifruit
Grapefruit
Mangoes
Blood Oranges
Cherries
Nectarines
Red Onions
Rhubarb
Papayas
Peaches
Persimmons
Rutabagas
Sweet Corn
Pomegranates
Potatoes
Radishes

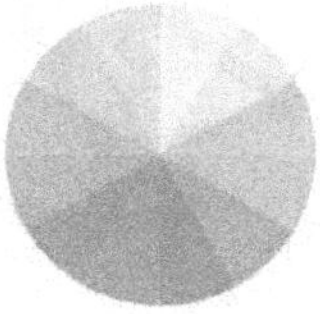

Butternut Squash
Apples
Beets
Orange Peppers
Chili Peppers
Cranberries
Red Peppers
Tangerines
Yellow Squash
Yellow Figs
Raspberries
Apricots
Tomatoes
Cantaloupe
Strawberries
Watermelon
Yellow Peppers

What makes up the colors of these fruits and vegetables?

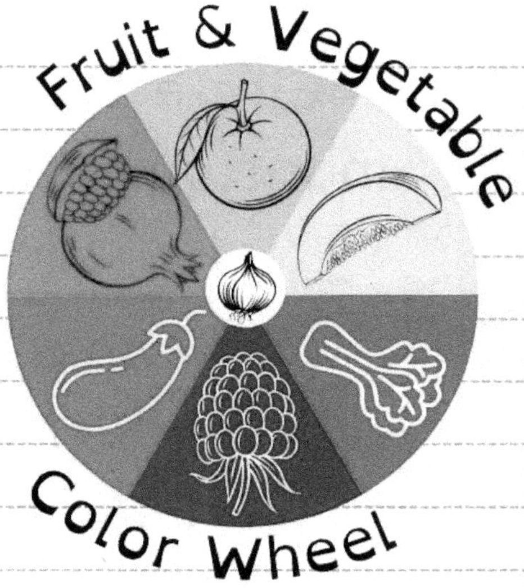

Which of these fruits and vegetables are some of your favorite foods?

How do they help keep your body healthy?

Circle the word if it is a fruit and underline the word if it is a vegetable. Include these on page 40.

Artichokes
Blackberries
Avocados
Eggplant
Cabbage
Cauliflower
Cucumber
Grapes
Pears
Green Beans
Potatoes
Elderberries
Prunes
White Peaches
Raisins
White Corn
Violet Carrots
White Nectarines
Zucchini

Black Currants
Mushrooms
Turnips
Blueberries
Leeks
Plums
Brussel Sprouts
Parsnips
Kale
Arugula
Asparagus
Green Peppers
Shallots
Kiwifruit
Onions
Limes
Garlic
Purple Potatoes
Okra

What makes up the colors of these fruits and vegetables?

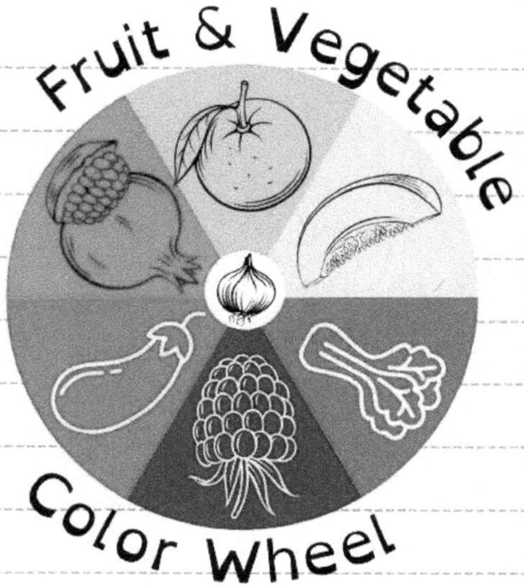

Which of these fruits and vegetables are some of your favorite foods?

How do they help keep your body healthy?

Draw your Fruit & Vegetable Color Wheel!

BRAIN Smoothie

Time To Recharge!

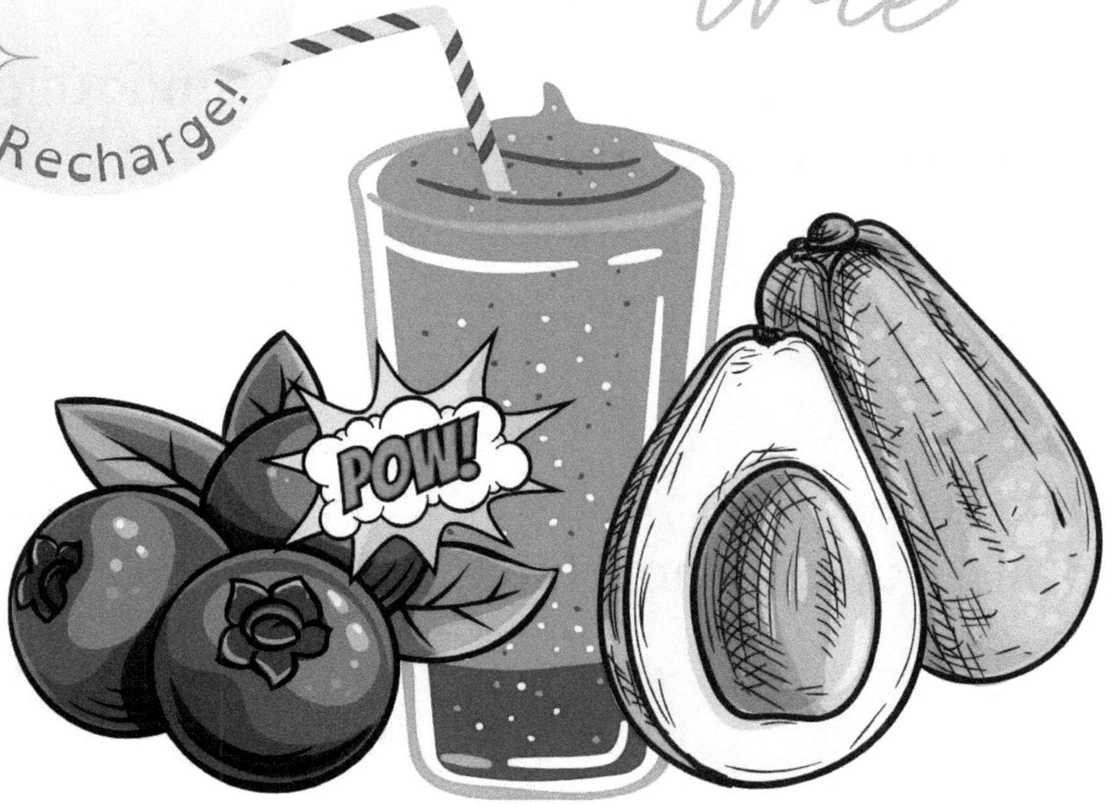

INGREDIENTS

Blueberries | Chia Seeds | Water | Banana | Honey | Berry Juice | Avocado

BLEND TOGETHER & ENJOY

3/4 cup Blueberries, frozen 1 Tablespoon Chia Seeds 1/2 cup Water 1 Banana, peeled	1 Tablespoon Honey 2 cups Berry Juice (cranberry, pomegranate, or other choice) 1/2 Avocado, peeled & no seed

Smoothie Reflection Time

Did you enjoy this recipe? Any changes?

Research and explain how this smoothie is good for your brain.

When would be a great time to drink this brain power smoothie?

Use as many descriptive words to explain the texture, flavor, consistency, etc. to someone who has never tried this smoothie before.

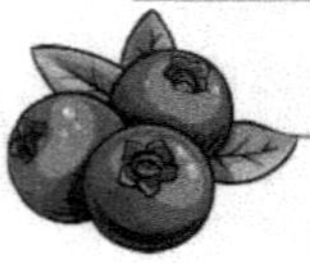

Rewrite your version of the recipe, making changes to quantities, steps, ingredients, or anything else you find fitting.

Recipe Name

Procedure

Yield

Cost

Time

Ingredients

How much would you charge for 16 oz?

What is your profit margin?

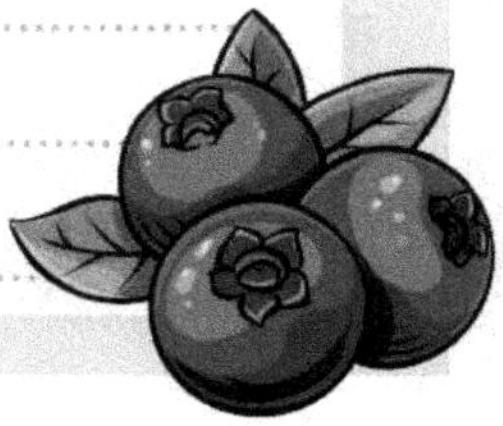

Fruit Math

Solve the equations by using the numbers each fruit represents. Remember to use the correct order of operation.

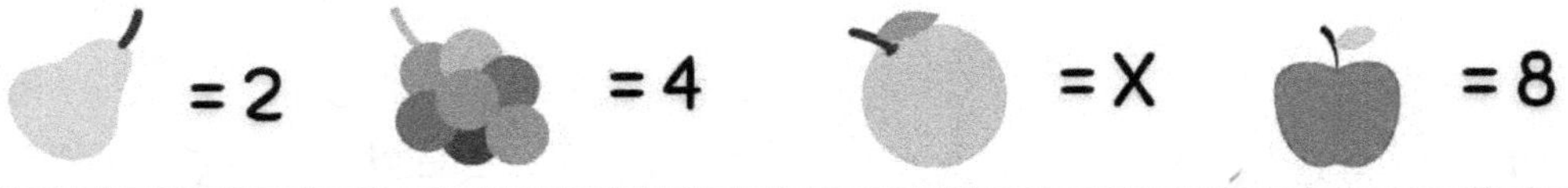

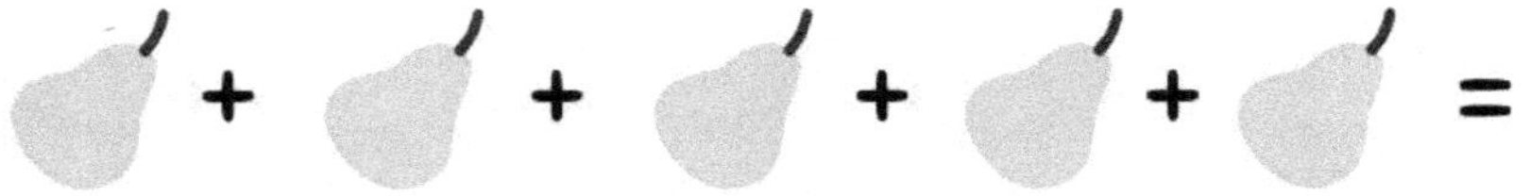

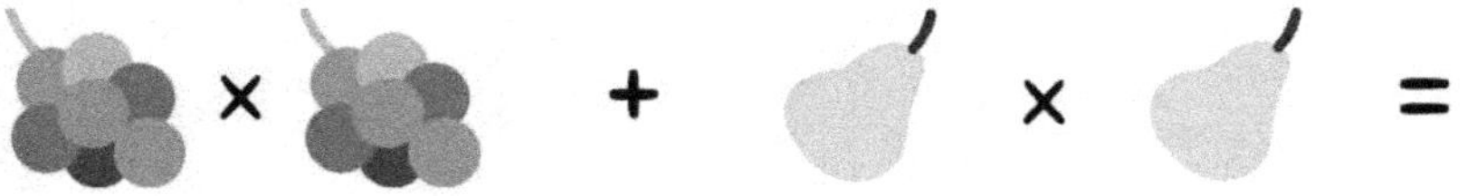

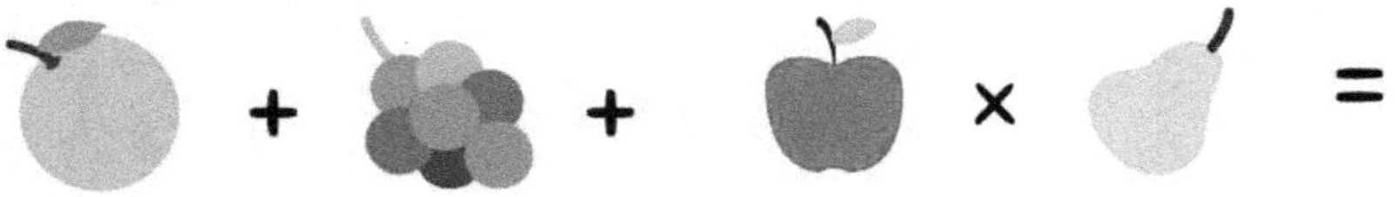

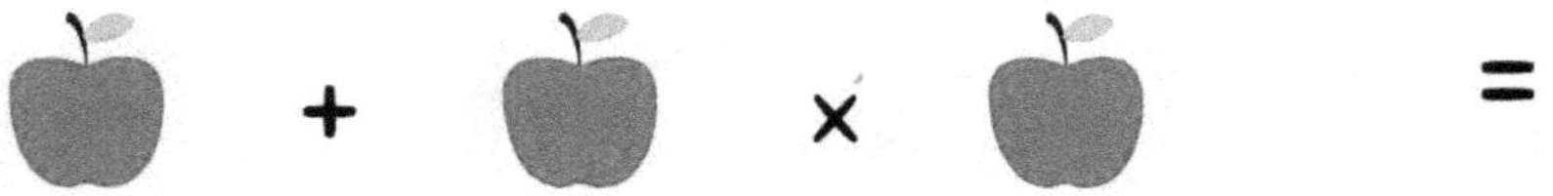

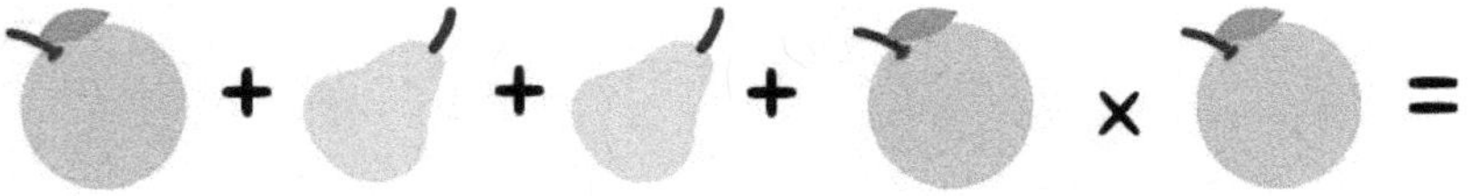

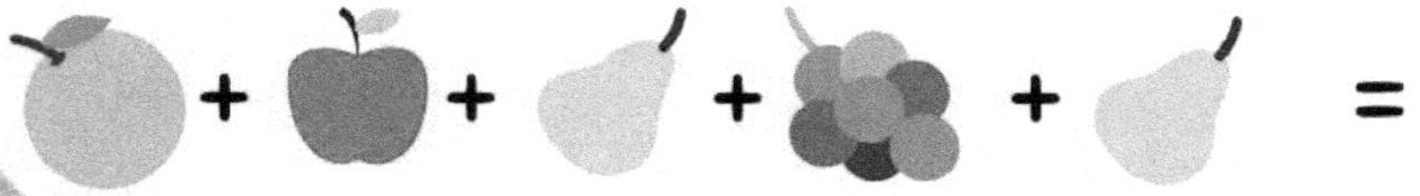

Fruit Math

Solve the equations by using the numbers each fruit represents. Remember to use the correct order of operation.

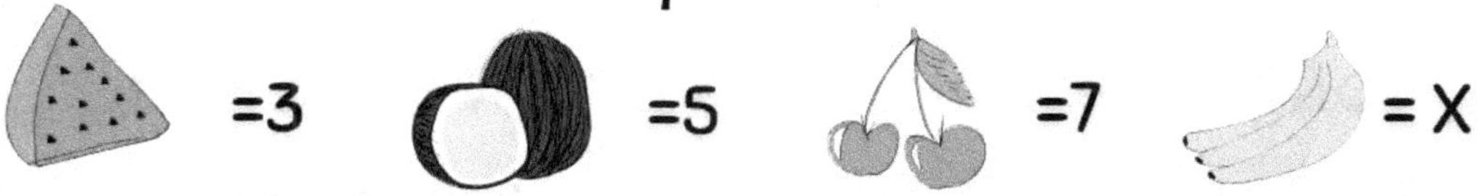

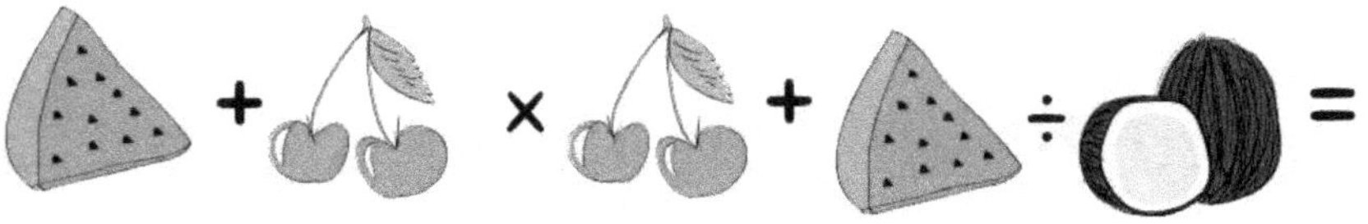

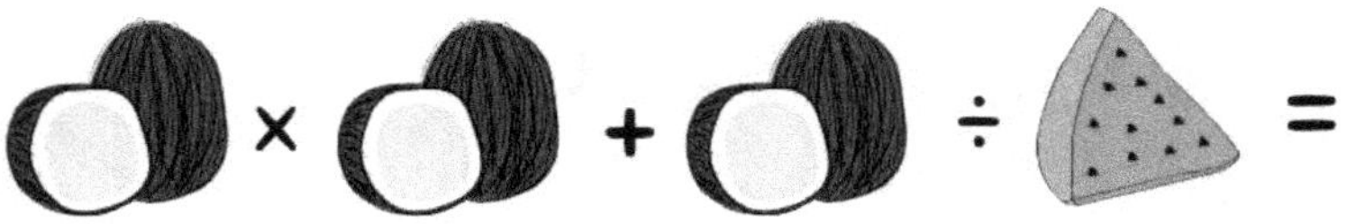

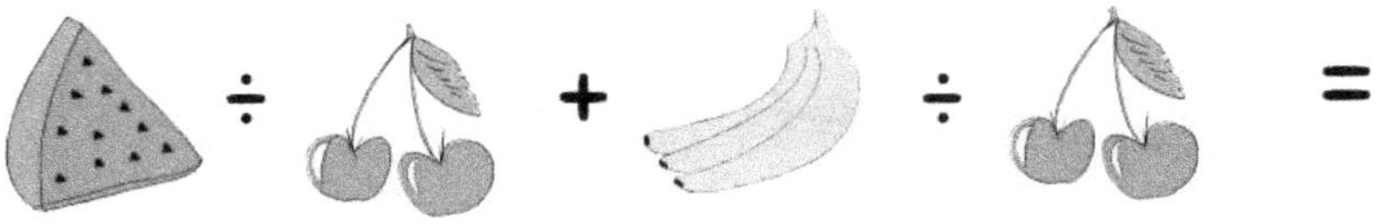

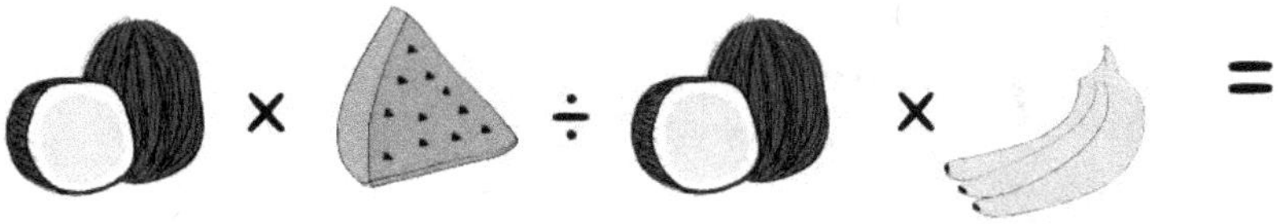

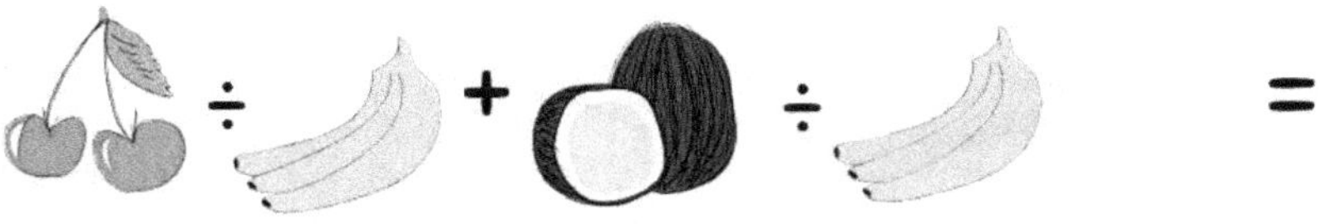

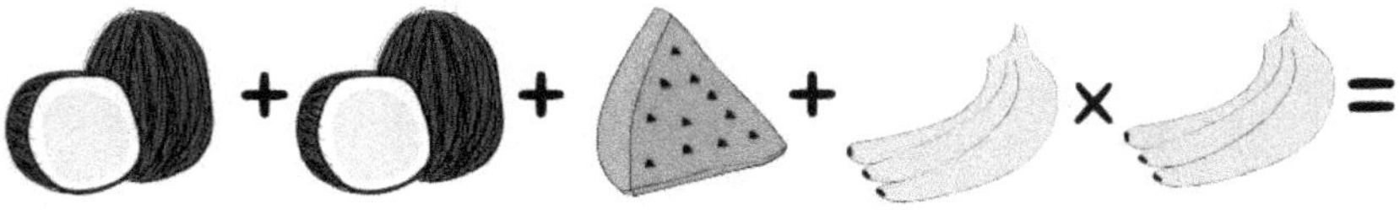

STILL LIFE DRAWING

Observe and freehand sketch a piece of your favorite fruit and vegetable. Consider your use of line, shape, and form.

Remember to have fun and to look up drawing tips, tricks, and some well known artists to get inspired!

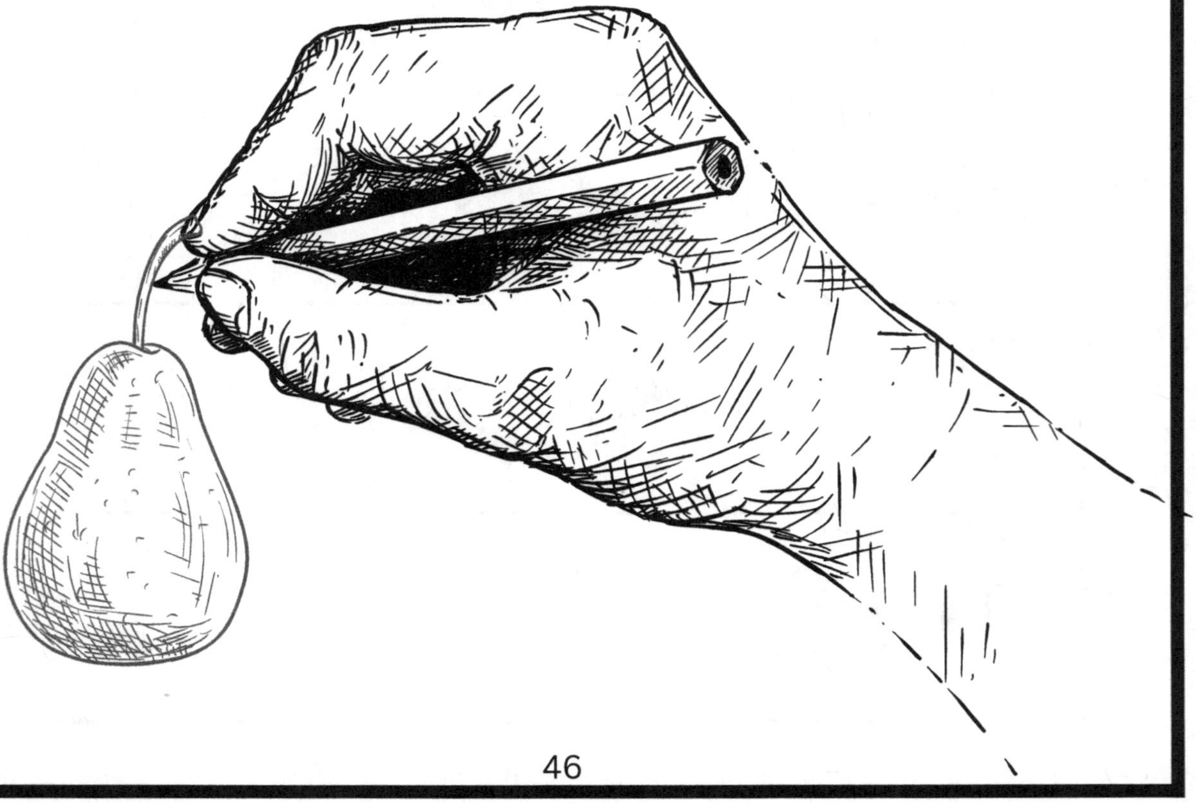

Favorite Fruit

Favorite Vegetable

Washing Fruits And Vegetables

From farm to grocery shelf, produce is exposed to a lot...
A great idea is to give them all a rinse before you take a bite!

From farm to grocery shelf, explain what produce is exposed to.

Do you clean your produce just before you eat it or when you bring it home. Explain your reasoning.

Clean Up

Whether you are eating produce from the Fifteen Clean or A Dozen Dirty Dozen list, choosing organic, non-GMO or GMO, all produce needs to be washed. Commercially grown and harvested fruits and vegetables have some amount of pesticide residue on them, even the organic options. What a great reason to wash your produce before you eat them! There are quite a few natural ways to wash your produce, find which method works best for you. On the next page, you can try a recipe at home to see if that method works for you. If not, the world wide web has an ample supply of alternative recipes for produce cleaning solutions!

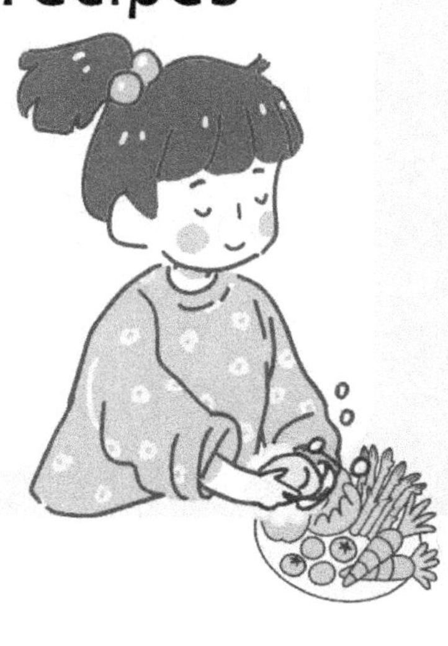

A Natural Cleaning Solution

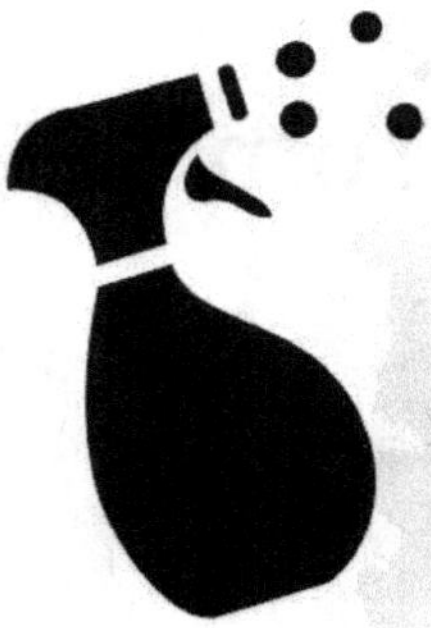

Ingredients:

1 cup White Vinegar
1/4 cup Apple Cider Vinegar
5 cups Filtered Water
10 drops Lemon Oil

Directions:

Mix all your ingredients in a large, non-metallic bowl. Add your produce and soak for 5-10 minutes. Be sure to gently scrub harder fruits and veggies, such as apples, and let your leafy greens and berries just soak (scrubbing would be too rough for them). Once the scrubbing or soaking time is up, rinse with filtered water and enjoy!

Remember, once your produce has been washed it is best to eat them as soon as possible, since washing them speeds up their oxidation and ripening process.

Pro Tip: Add this solution to a spray bottle.

Did you find the natural cleaning solution to be effective at cleaning your produce? Why or why not?

If you have another method, recipe, or searched something online, share your findings below.

You only have 1/8 cup of Apple Cider Vinegar for the recipe. Rewrite the ingredients to adjust for the vinegar.

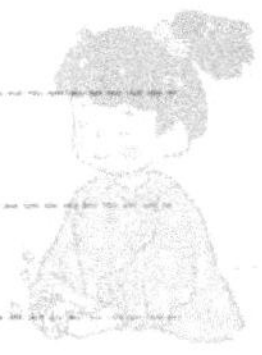

Some spinach and other leafy greens are packaged and labeled "triple washed." Explain this process and if it is ready to eat.

Research and explain how commercially harvested produce is washed.

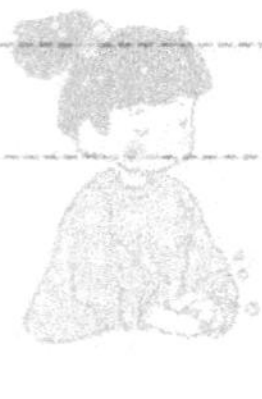

Fifteen Clean

Research and describe what the clean fifteen produce means.

Practice your cursive handwriting skills!

Are these studies on produce right off the shelf or on cleaned produce? Explain the testing process.

Fifteen Clean

Label and color.

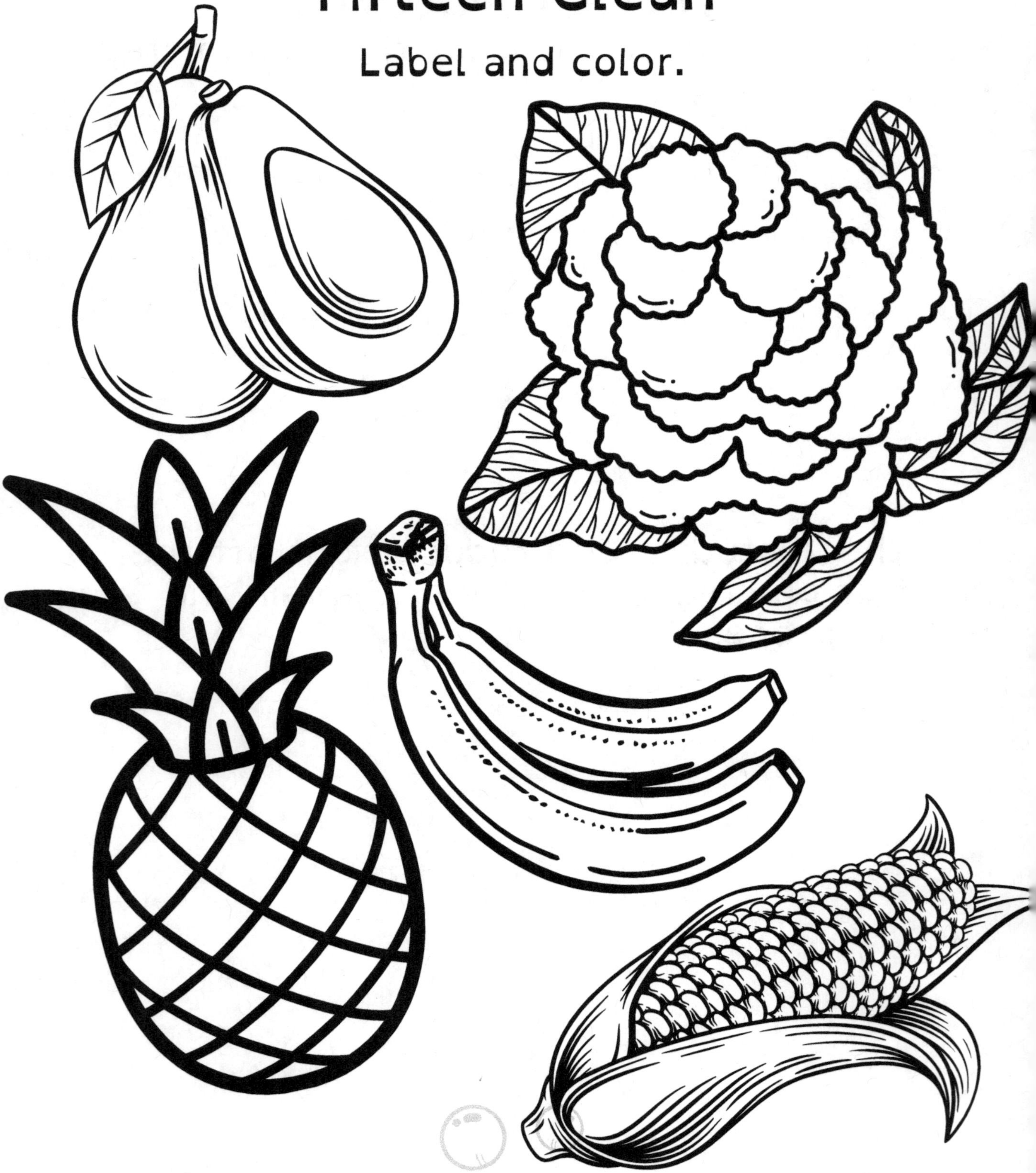

- Results are from EWG 2025 tests.

Fifteen Clean

Label and color.

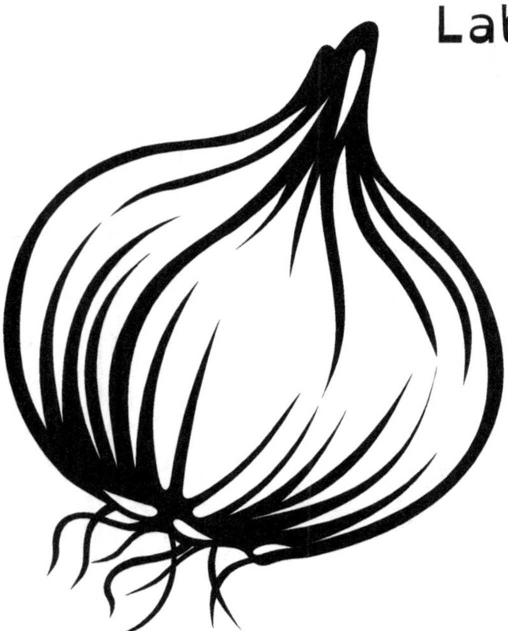

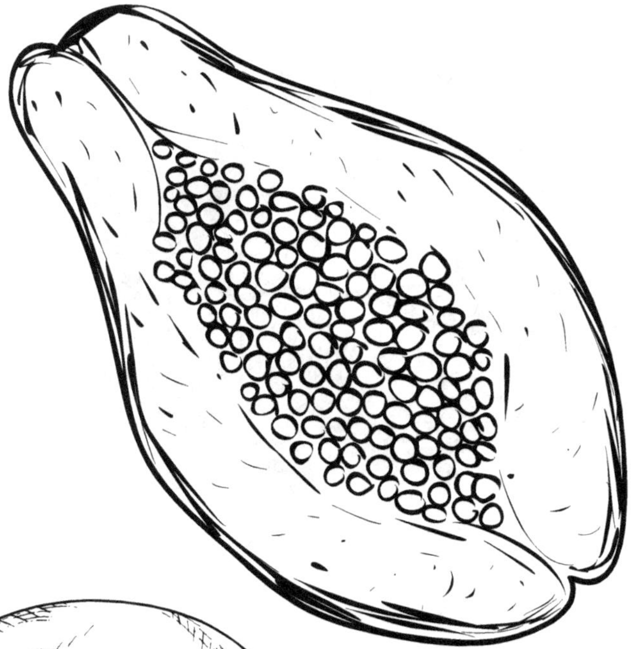

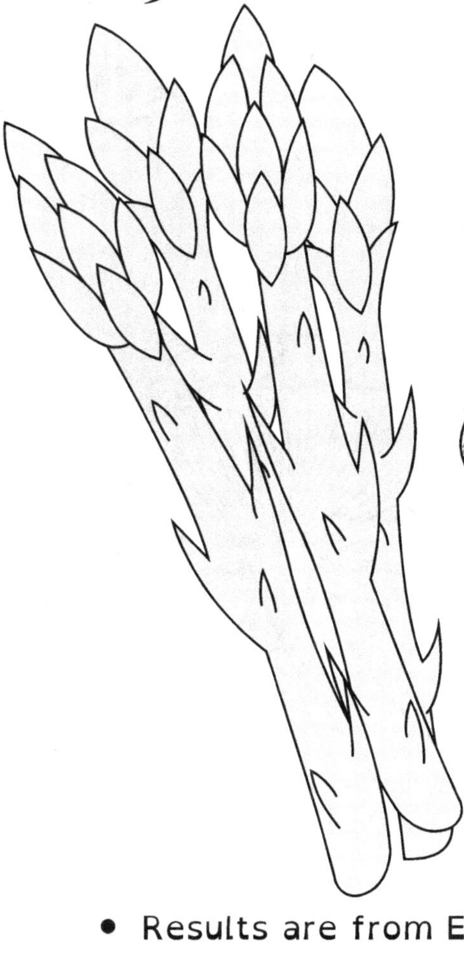

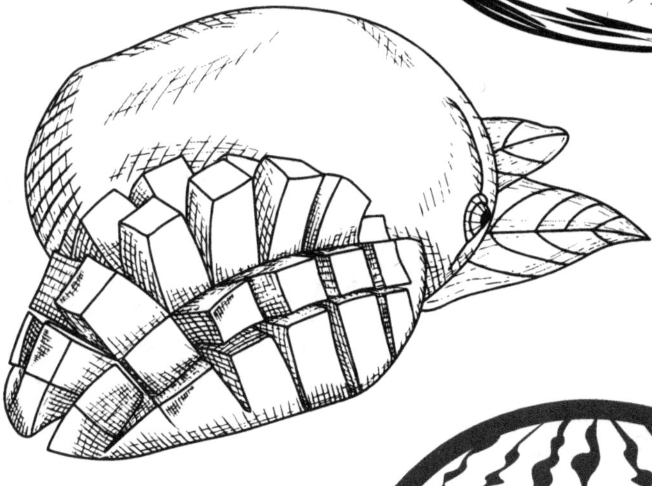

- Results are from EWG 2025 tests.

Fifteen Clean

Label and color.

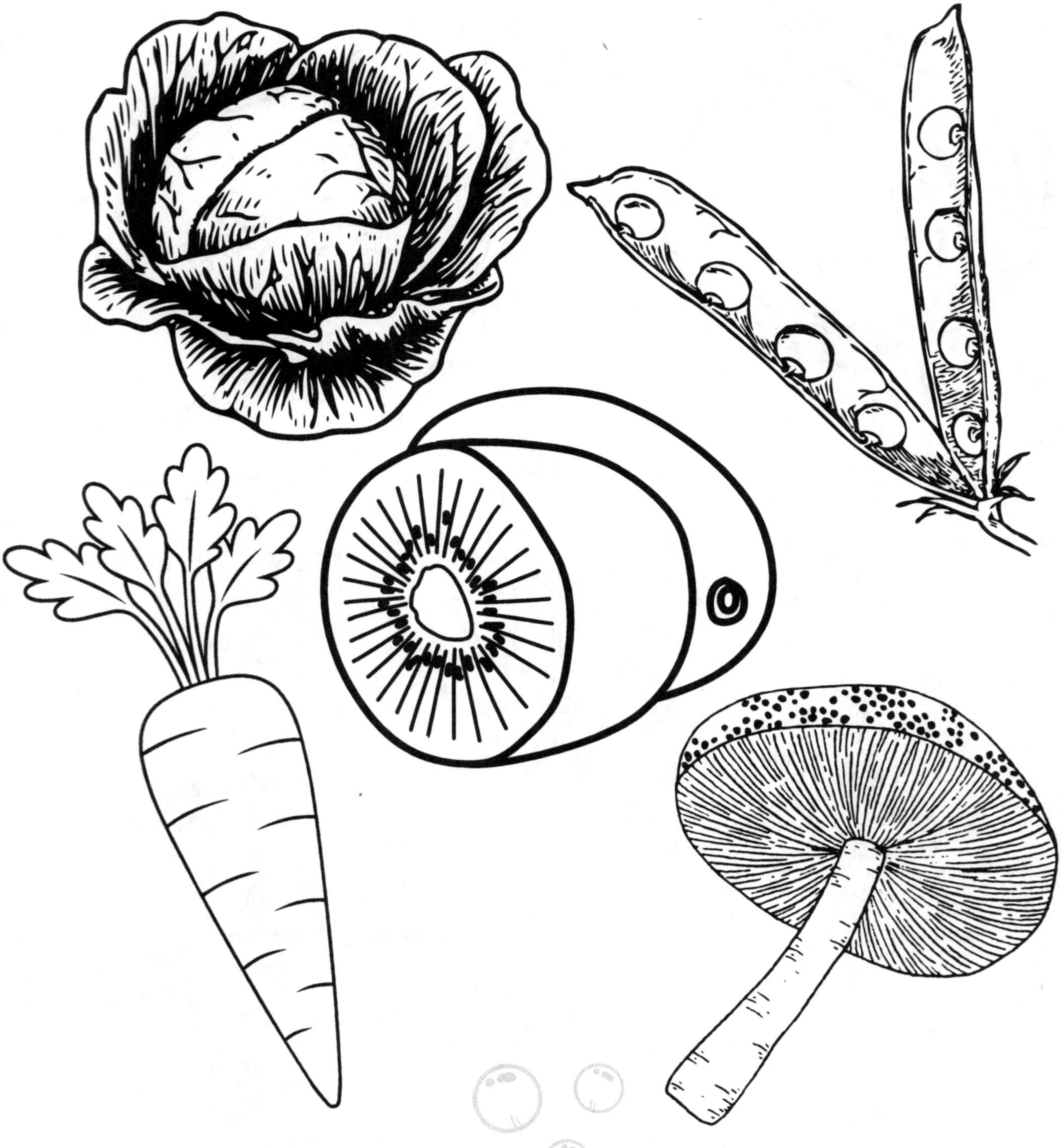

- Results are from EWG 2025 tests.

A Dozen Dirty

Research and describe what the dirty dozen produce means.

What chemicals or pesticides are used on these 'dirty' fruits and vegetables? Explain the dangers of those pesticides.

A Dozen Dirty

Label and color.

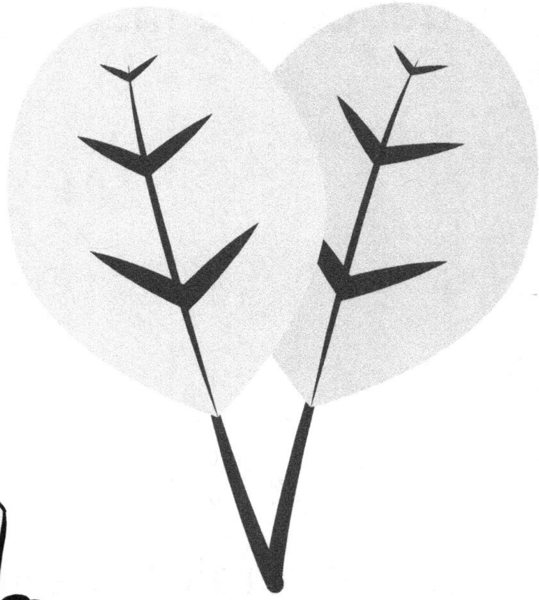

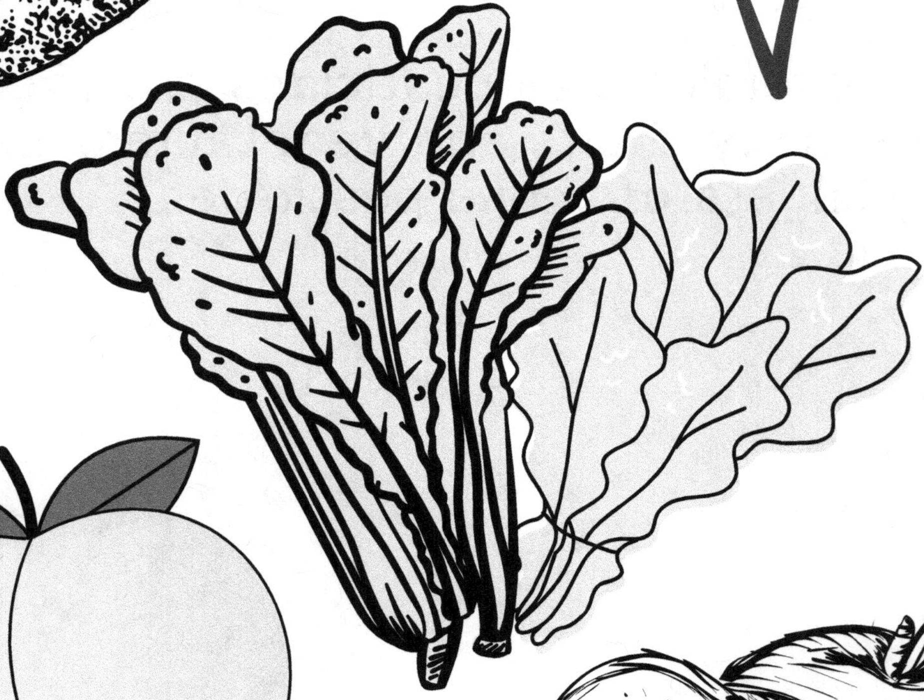

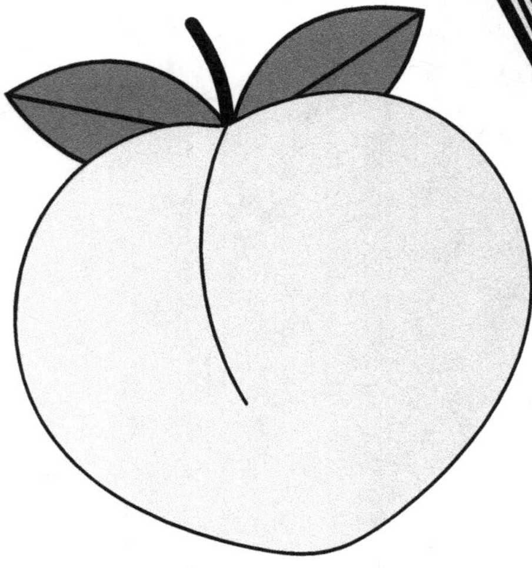

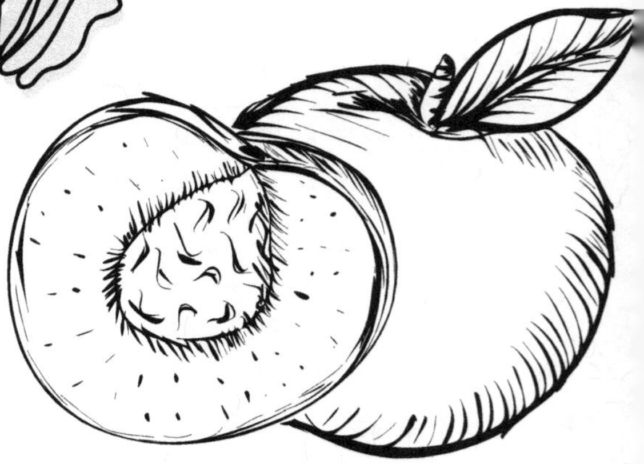

- Results are from EWG 2025 tests.

A Dozen Dirty

Label and color.

- Results are from EWG 2025 tests.

Observation Questions

Take a look at the Fifteen Clean foods and then take a look at A Dozen Dirty food list. Are there some things you see in common or different?

Explain how characteristics in produce can help you choose clean, low pesticide fruits and vegetables.

What about dehydrated foods, such as raisins, are these free of pesticides?

What about processed foods that contain strawberries, such as strawberry ice cream or strawberry jam, would these contain pesticides? Explain.

What about the organic options?

What about all the other fruits and vegetables that are not on the Fifteen Clean or A Dozen Dirty list, are they free of pesticides? Explain.

Describe several ways to make sure you are eating clean fruits and vegetables.

Research and write about the history of pesticides. When they became, why and what effects have they had?

Fruit Salad

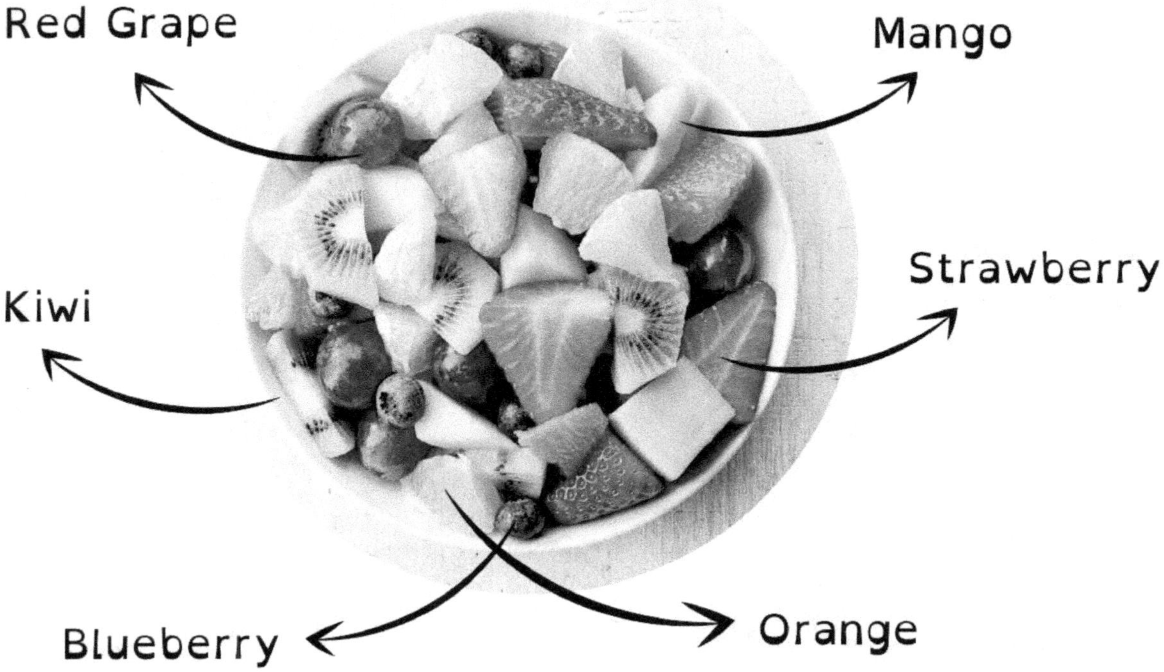

Which fruits would you recommend organic? Explain.

What other ingredients and superfoods could you add? (Like yogurt, granola, etc.)

Name some of the health benefits of this salad.

Circle the food that should be purchased in the organic section of your grocery store.

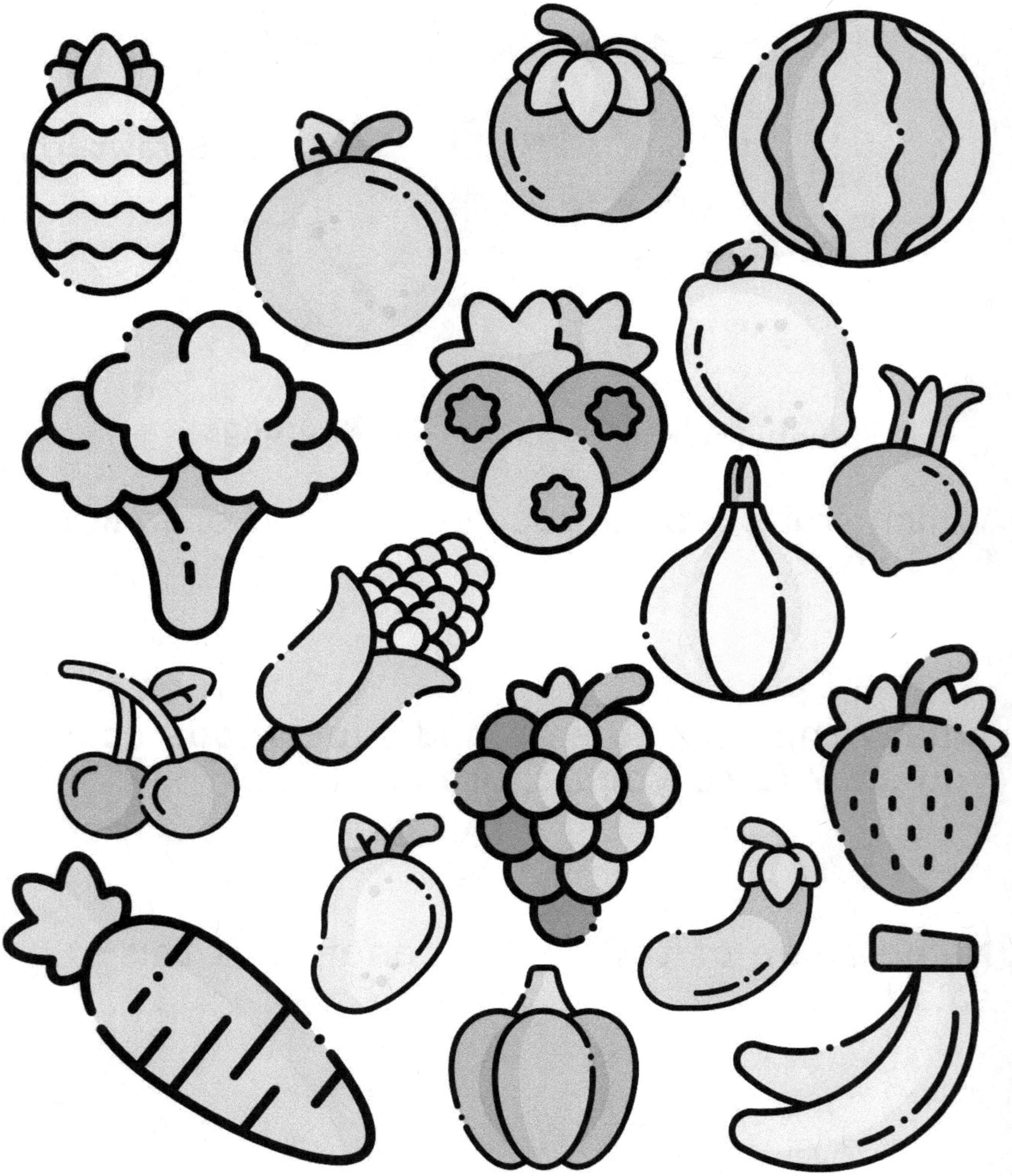

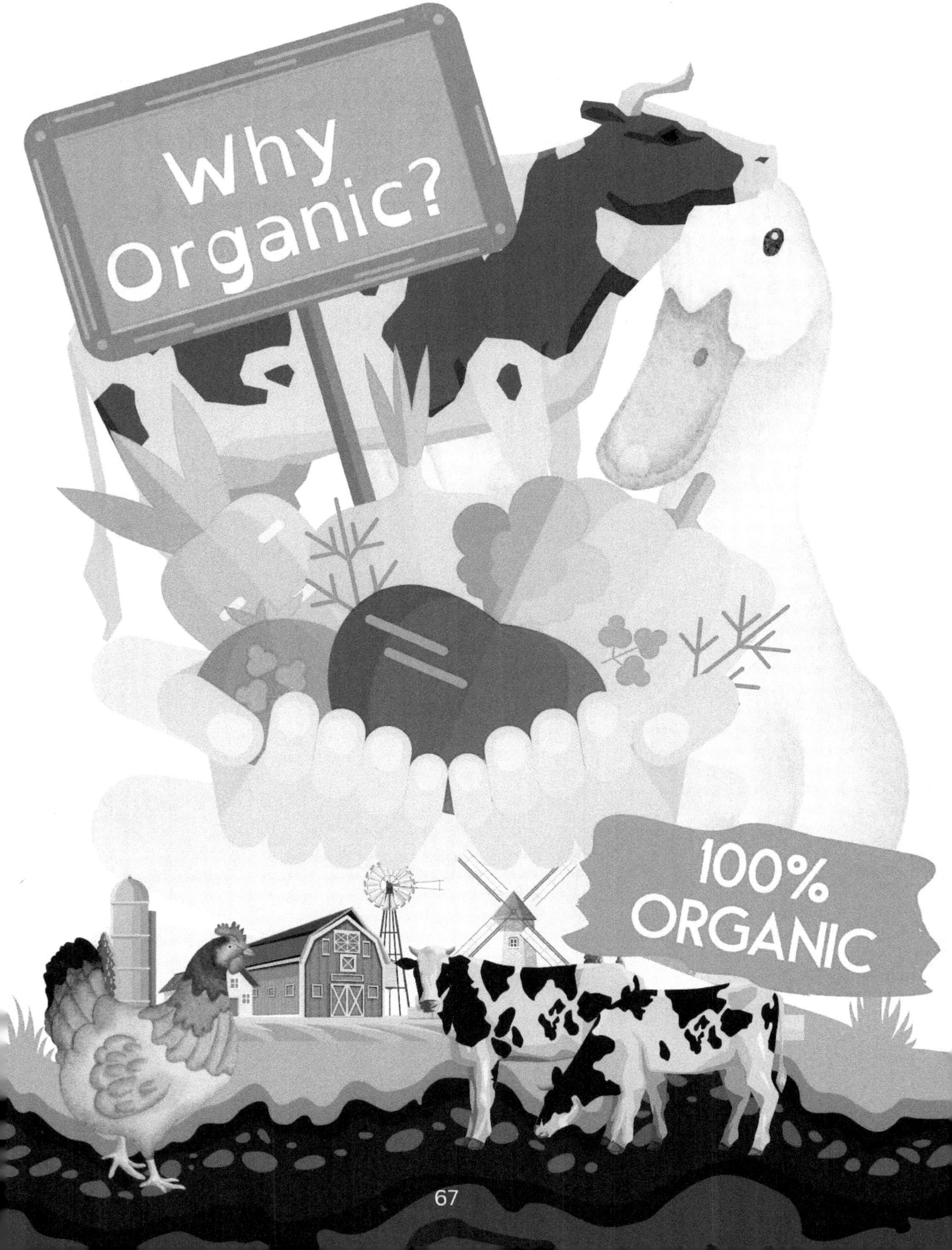
Why
Organic?
100%
ORGANIC

What Does Organic Mean?

We used to not have to think about food being anything but organic, but with agricultural changes, it is important to be informed about what you eat and where it comes from. Research and write what organic meat, eggs, dairy, grains, fruits and vegetables mean.

Practice your cursive handwriting skills!

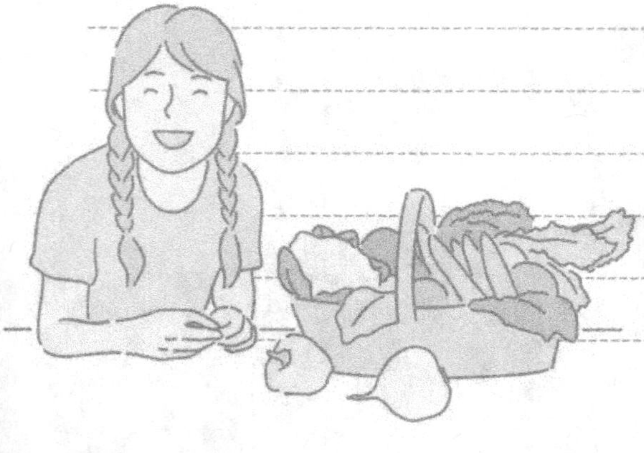

Research and describe organic regenerative farming. Explain how this can benefit our planet.

Describe the history of organic farming. Is this similar or different in other countries?

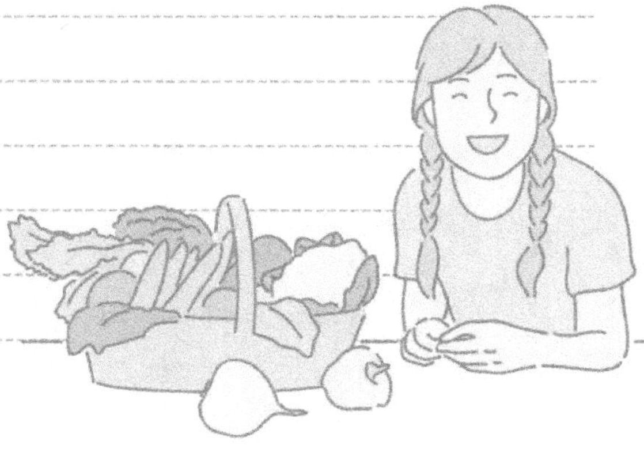

What does GMO mean?

Explain the positive aspects of GMO.

What are the problems with GMO?

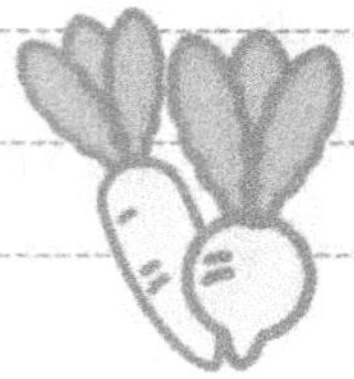

Place the phrases under the correct column.

ORGANIC	NON-ORGANIC

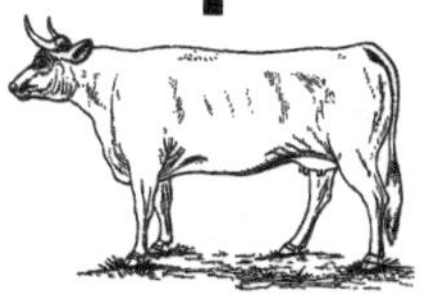

- Cannot have any GMO ingredients.
- May use sewage sludge for fertilizer.
- May contain genetically modified organisms.
- May contain growth hormones.
- Food may have been irradiated.
- Must not contain more than 5% of non-organic content.
- Soil must not have had any synthetic fertilizers on it for at least 3 years.
- Animal living and grazing conditions are to be close to natural living conditions.

Define Irradiate:

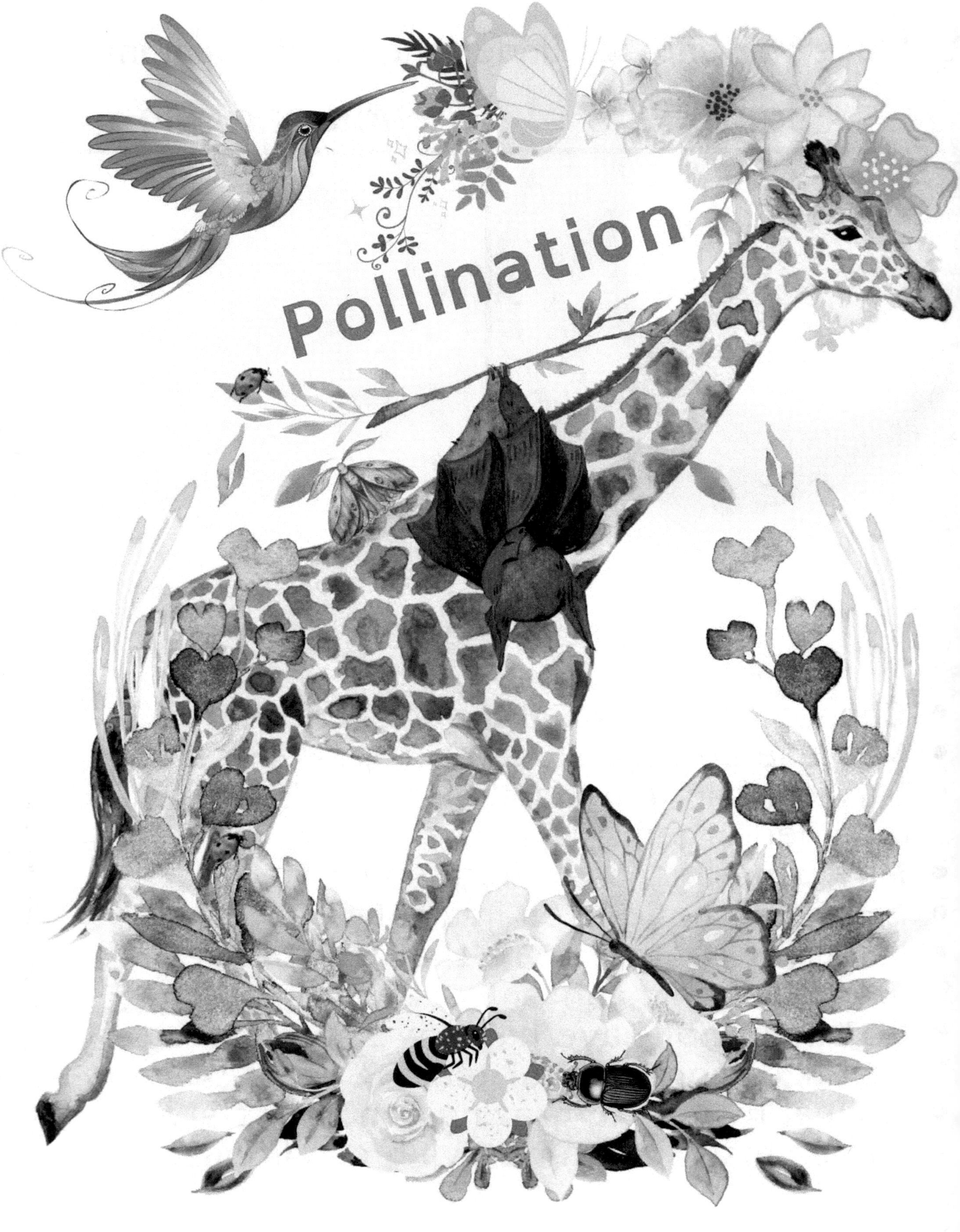
Pollination

What is pollen?

What is pollination?

How do the farmers and the pollinators work together in food production?

Practice your cursive handwriting skills!

Name as many pollinators as you can.
Put a star next to the ones you see around your home and community.

Do all plants need flowers to be pollinated?

Explain self-pollinating plants.

Has GMO plants effected pollinators?

Explain some risks that pollinators are experiencing.

What can be done to help?

Can planting local and native flowering plants help? Explain.

How can certified organic foods be helpful for the environment and the pollinator too?

Go through some of the fruits and vegetables in this book, and discover which ones need to be pollinated. Write them below.

STILL LIFE DRAWING

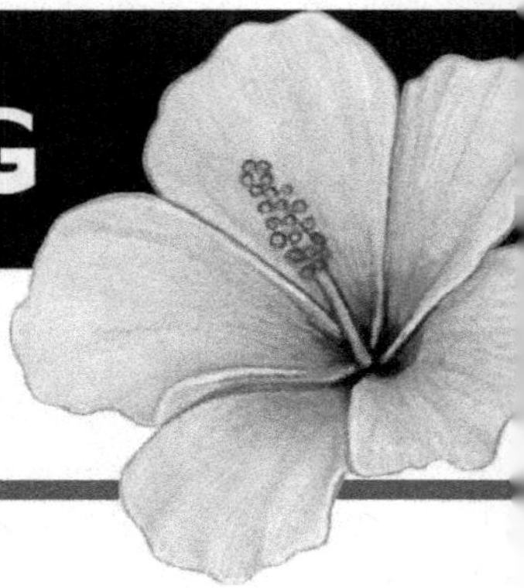

Sketch your favorite flower and pollinator.

A Flower's Journey

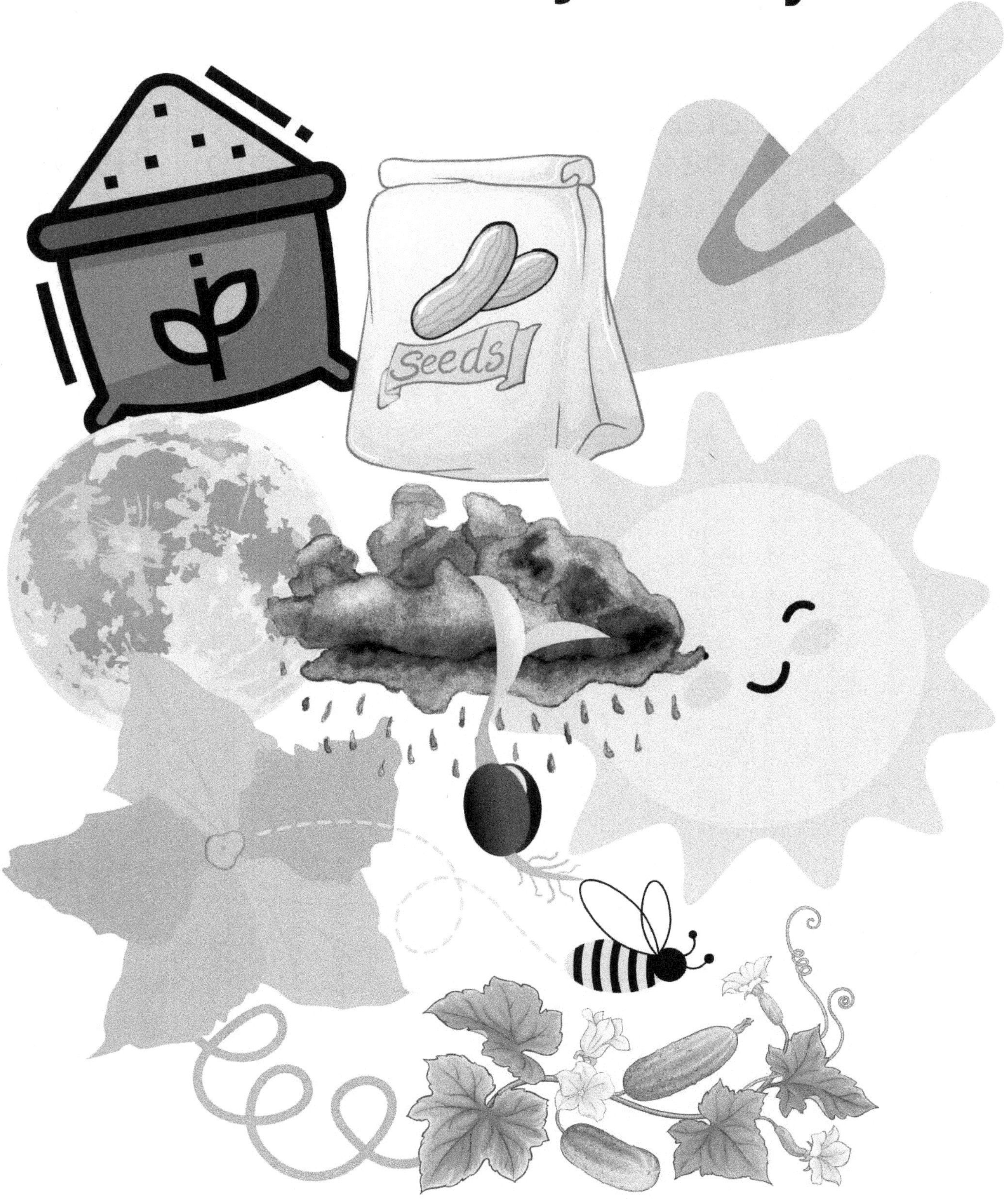

Write a story, describing the process from seed, flower, pollination, to fruit. Use the pictures on the previous page for reference. Research more details, such as how long from pollinating does the fruit start to grow. Have fun and be creative!

Practice your cursive handwriting skills!

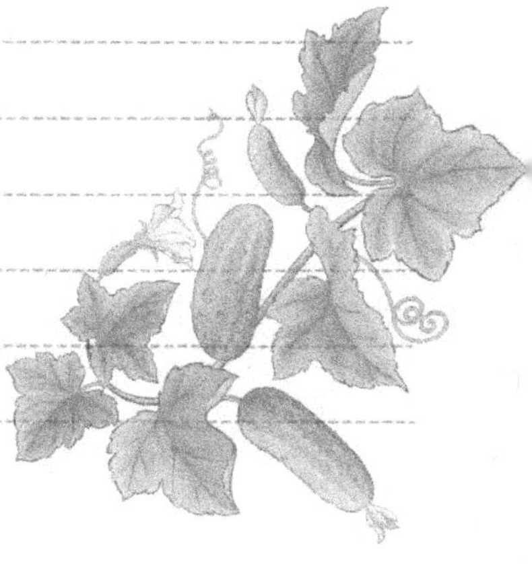

CUCUMBER *Pucker*

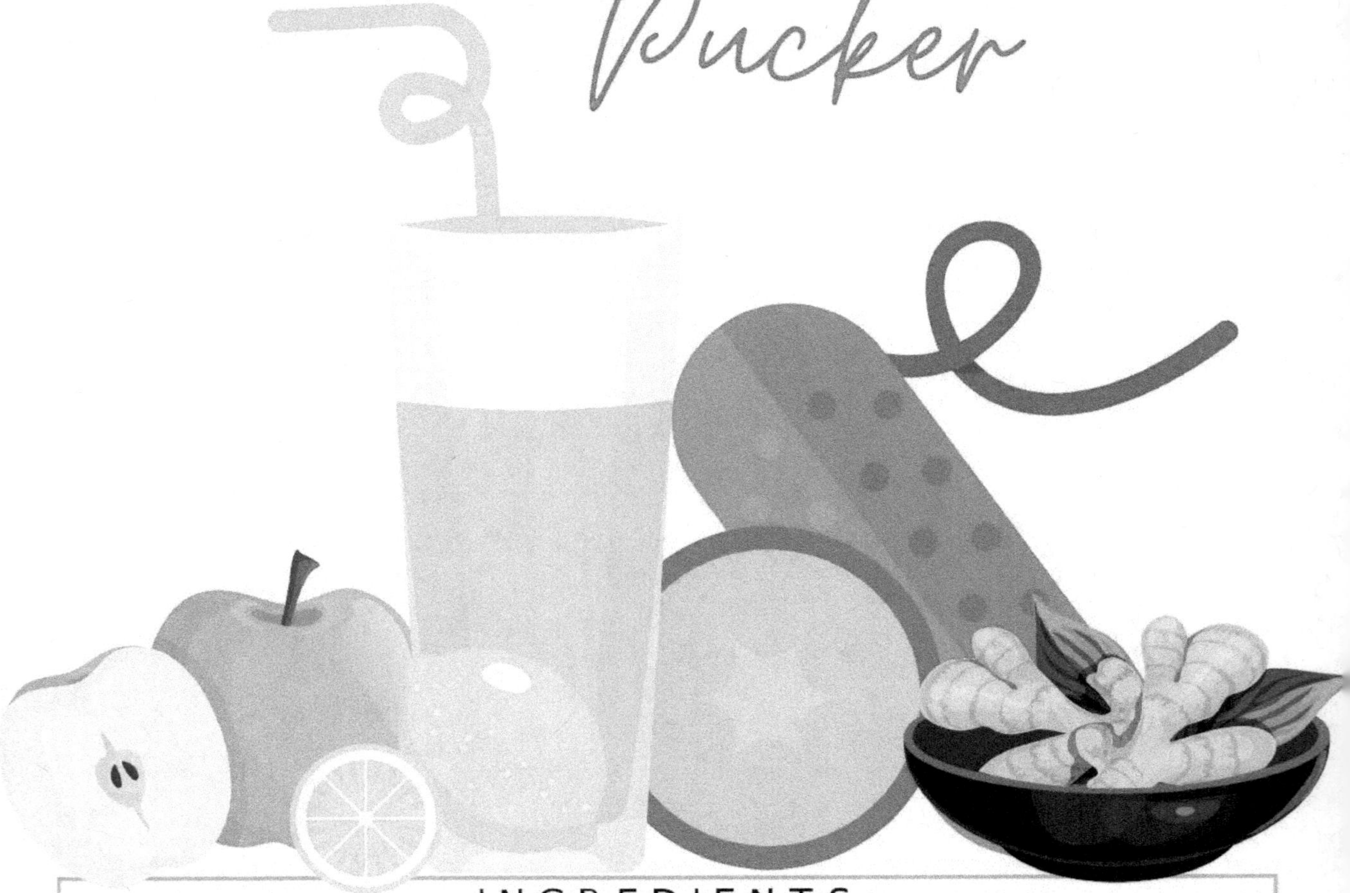

INGREDIENTS

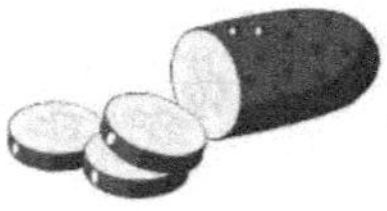
Cucumber

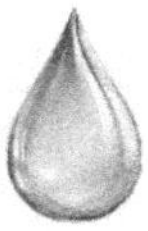
Water

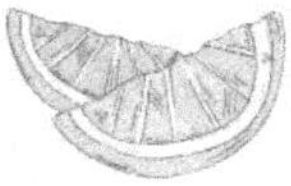
Lemon Juice

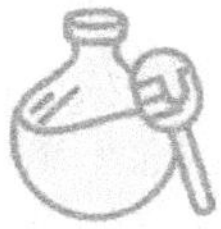
Honey

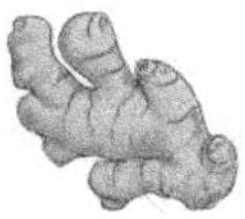
Ginger

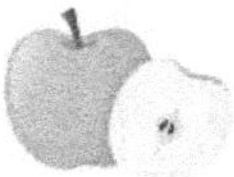
Green Apple

BLEND TOGETHER & ENJOY

1 Cucumber 1 1/2 cups water 2 Tablespoons Lemon Juice	1-2 Tablespoons Honey 1/2 teaspoon Ginger 1 Green Apple

Smoothie Reflection Time

Did you enjoy this recipe?

Did you use anything organic?
Did you plant any of the cucumber or lemon seeds?

What would you like to eat with this drink?

Use as many descriptive words to tell someone about your ice drink.

If you were to buy this drink at a smoothie stand, how much would you pay?
How would your presentation of this drink be unique and memorable, if you were to sell it in your smoothie stand?

About Some Measurements

Cucumbers range in many dimensions, some can be 10 inches, while others 3 inches. Not one is exactly like the other. This same idea can be applied with many fruits and veggies. The Cucumber Icey recipe calls for one cucumber and half an apple, which sizes, amounts, or weights worked for you?

Find the combination of measurements that tastes the best for you and rewrite the recipe on the next page. To be more precise about measurements, you are welcome to weigh out your ingredients with a scale. Make any adjustments to customize your drink recipe.

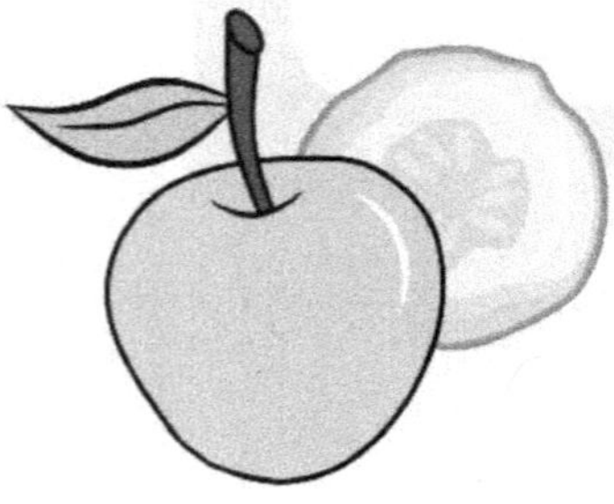

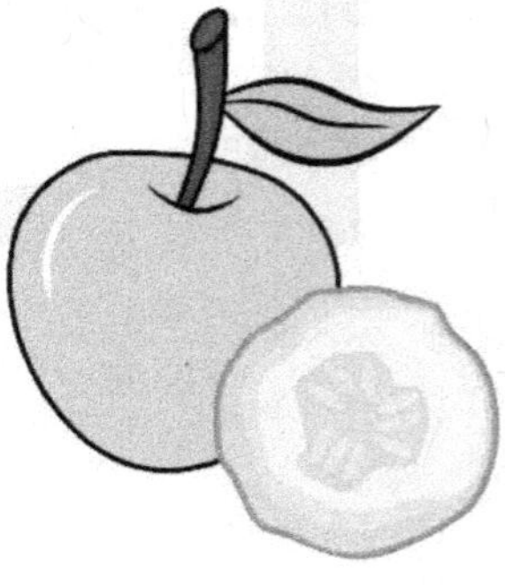

Rewrite your version of the recipe, making changes to quantities, steps, ingredients, or anything else you find fitting.

Recipe Name

Procedure

Yield

Cost

Time

Ingredients

How much would you charge for 16 oz?

What is your profit margin?

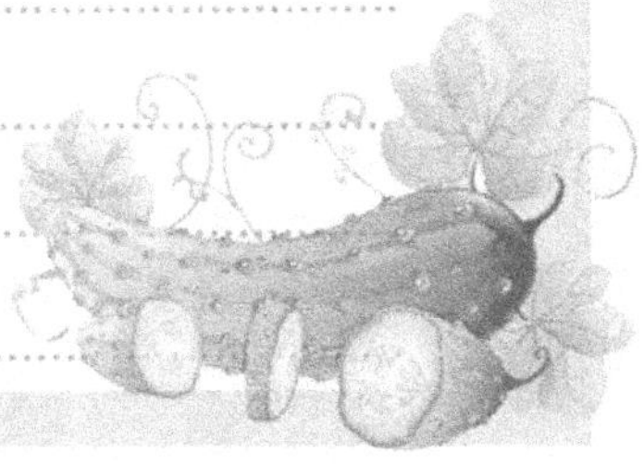

Mother Earth provides us with all our amazing foods...

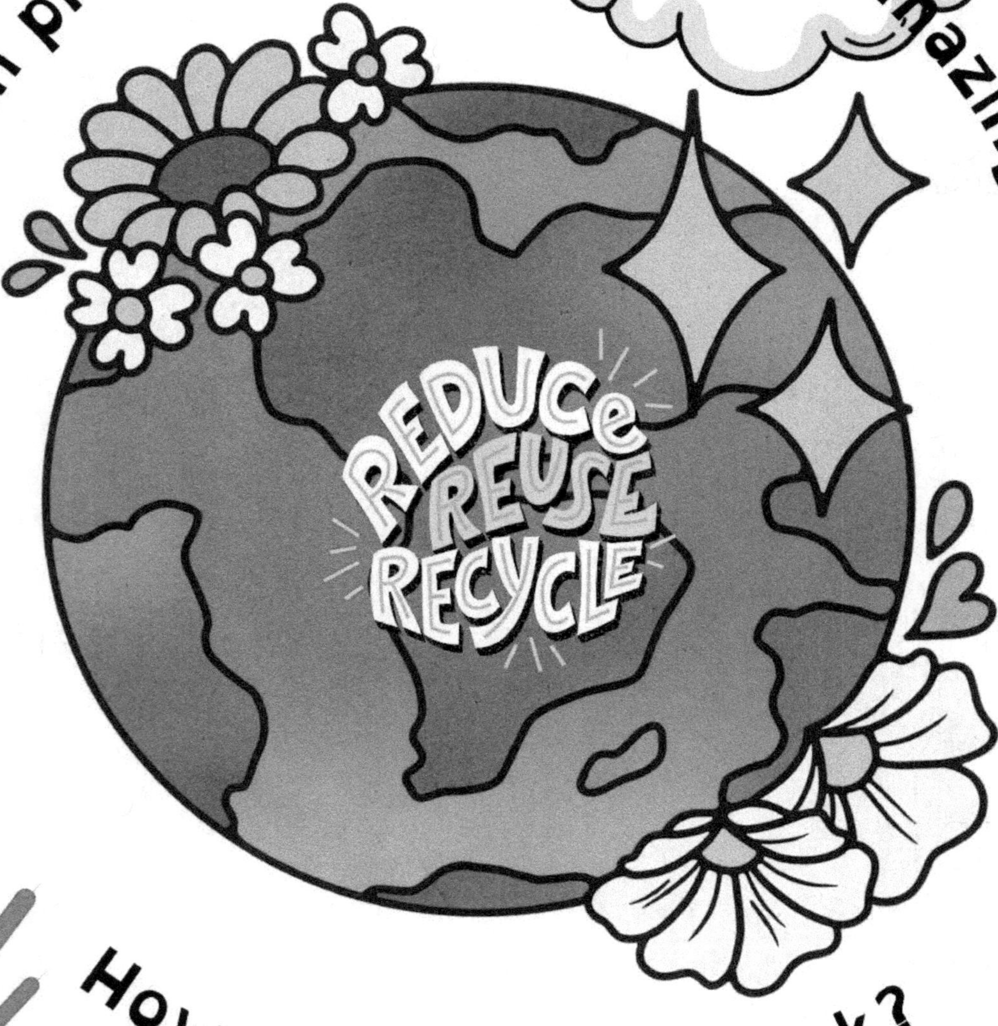

How can we give back?

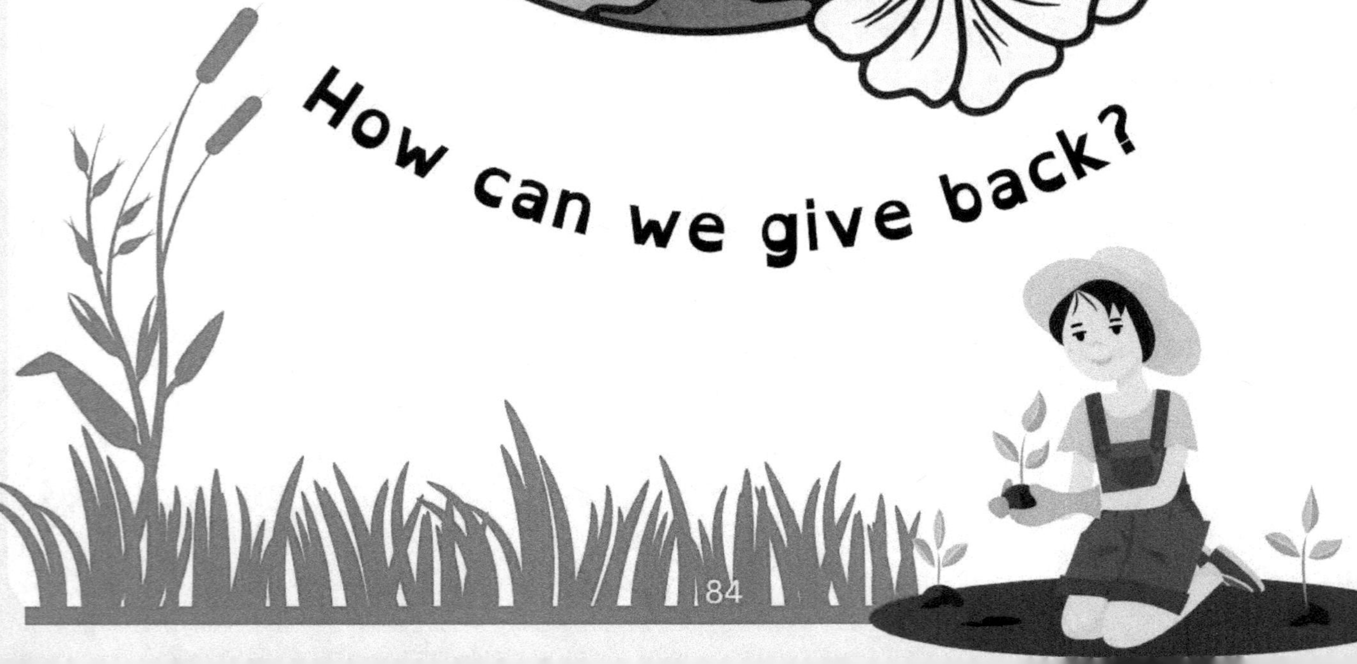

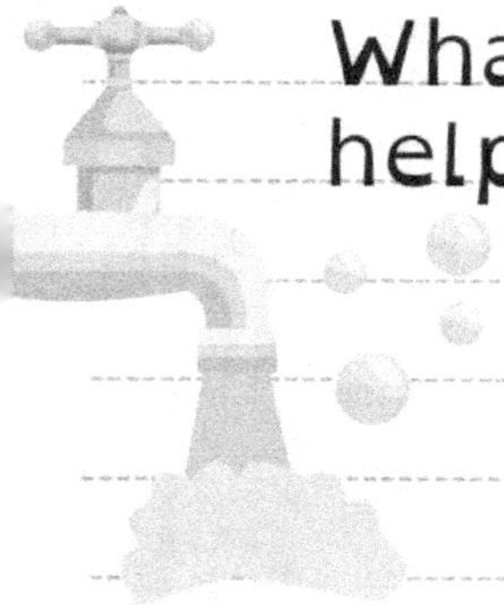

What are some things that you can do to help our planet stay healthy and clean?

I can help our planet by **reducing:**

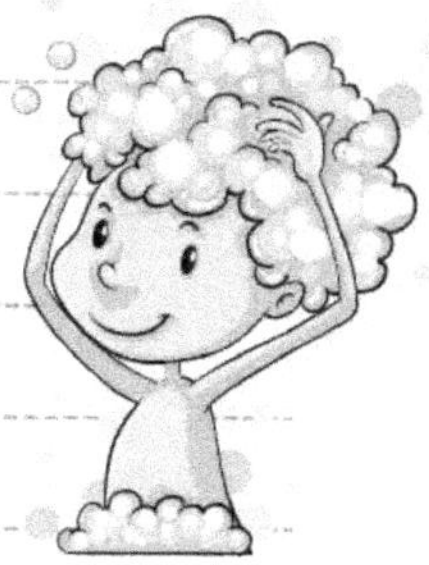

I can help our planet by **reusing/repurposing:**

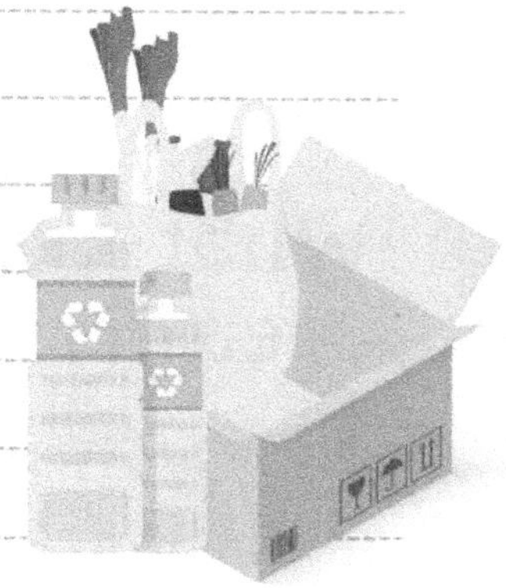

I can help our planet by **recycling:**

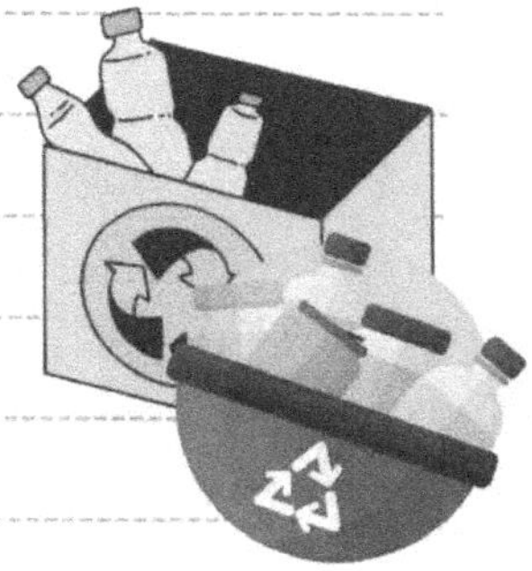

MORE IDEAS

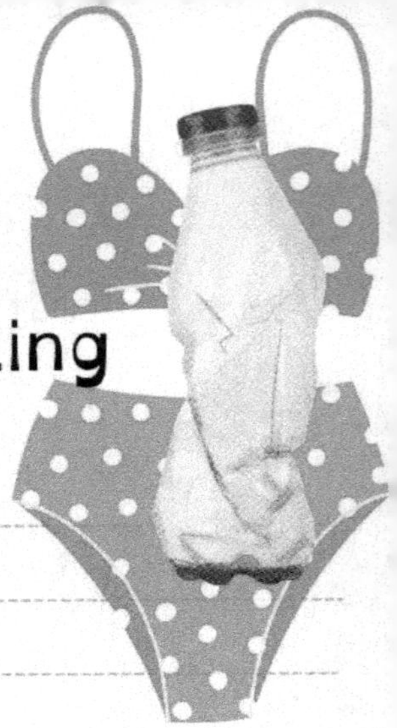

Swimsuits can be made out of plastic bottles! Start researching how recycling can recreate. Write what you find.

What kind of recycling is available in your area?

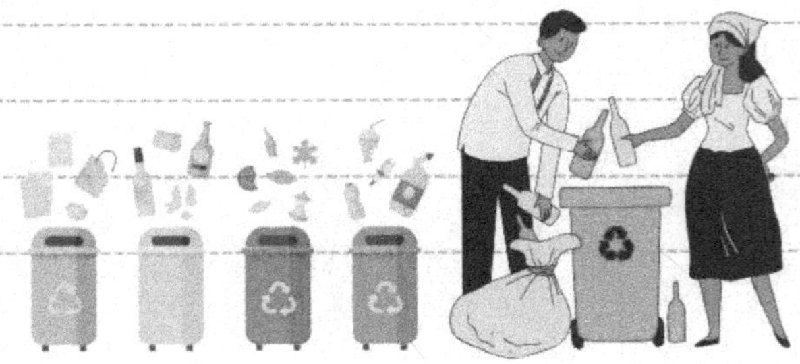

The Recycle King

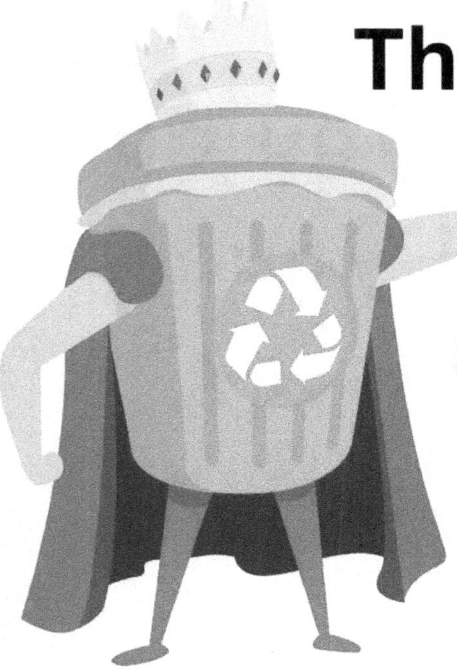

Get creative and find another purpose for something you would have thrown out in the trash or recycling bin. Have fun and recreate!

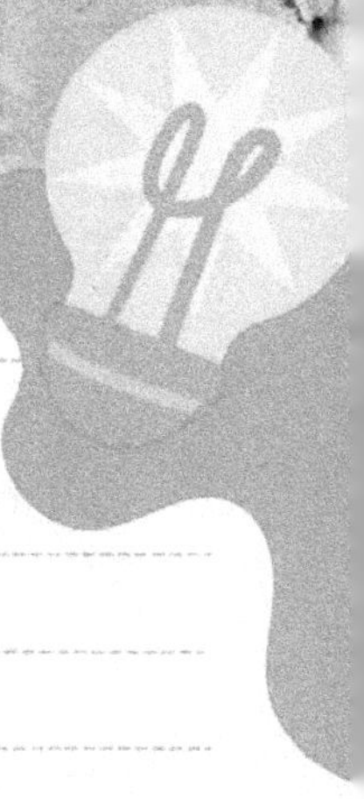

Build a fort with a cardboard box. Make a card, book, or journal using paper or cardboard from packages (cereal boxes work great).

What do you do with all your food waste?

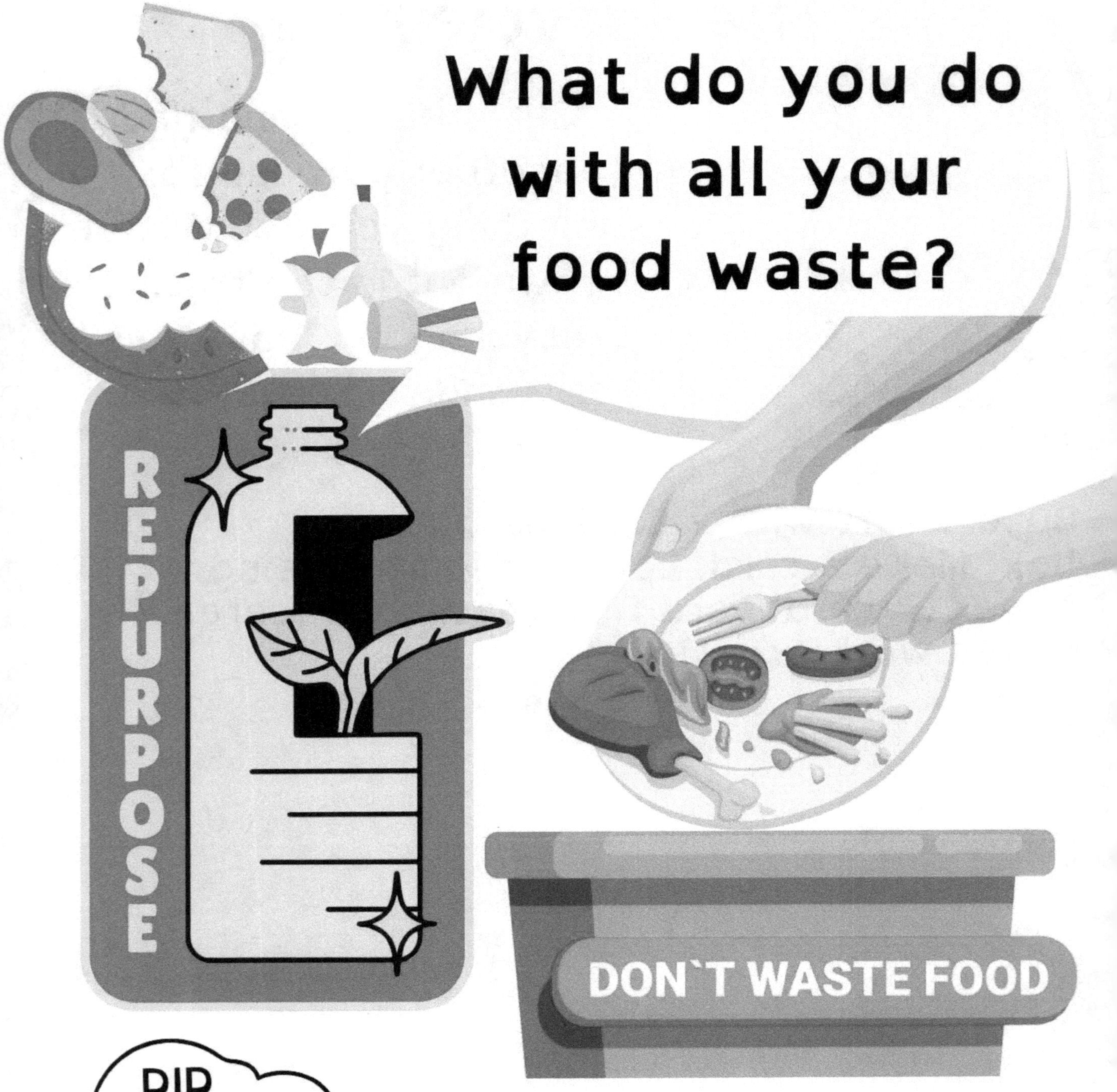

DID YOU KNOW?

In the USA, nearly 40% of all food is wasted. Research why and write a few solutions.

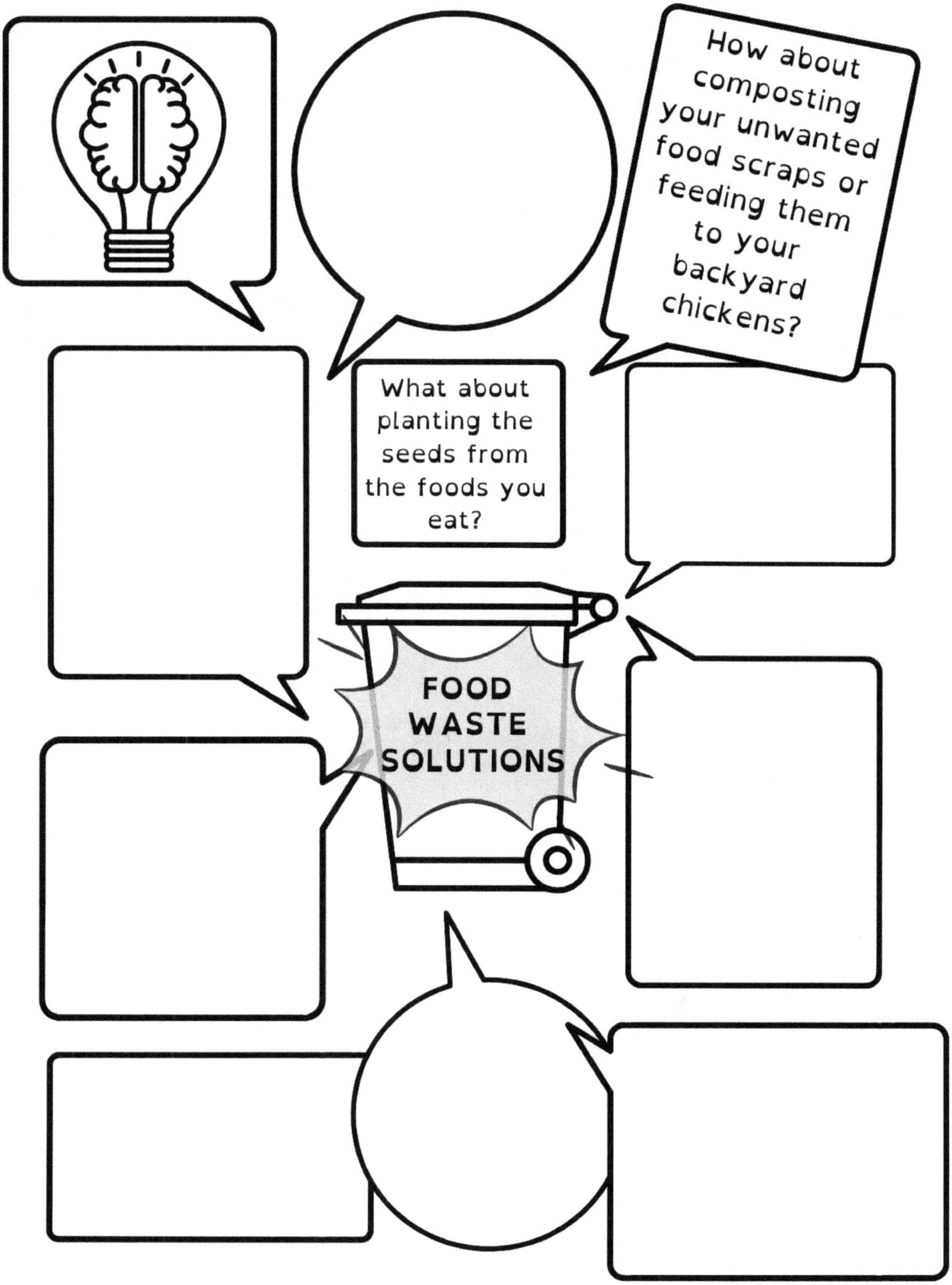
How about composting your unwanted food scraps or feeding them to your backyard chickens?
What about planting the seeds from the foods you eat?
FOOD WASTE SOLUTIONS

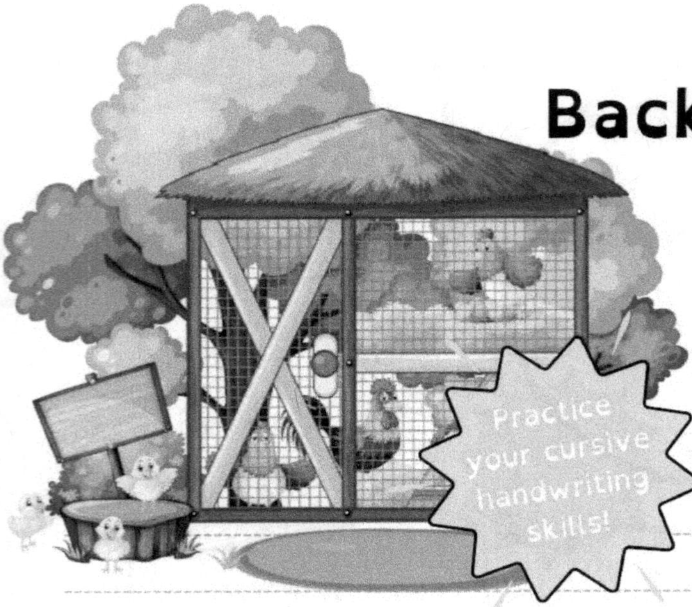

Backyard Chickens

Research and list some amazing benefits of having chickens in your yard.

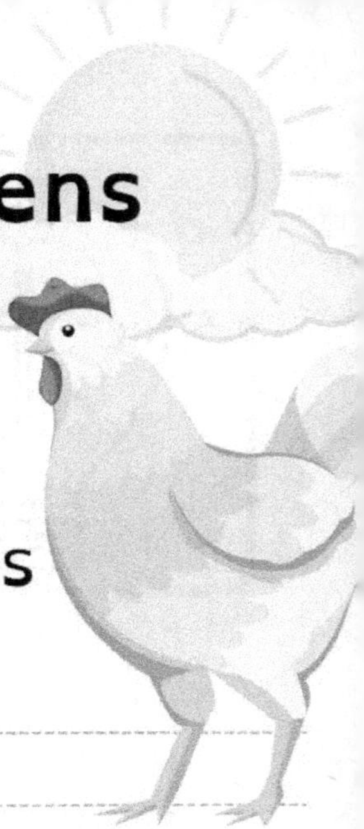

The Appeal In Peels

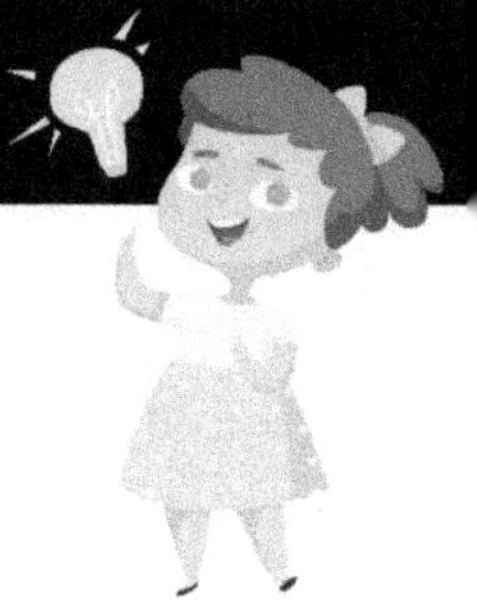

Research and list several different things you can do with these food leftovers.

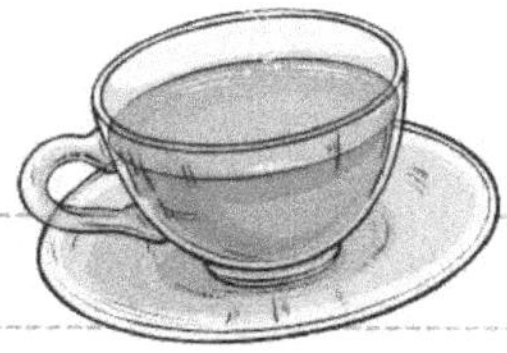

Onion and Garlic Skins:

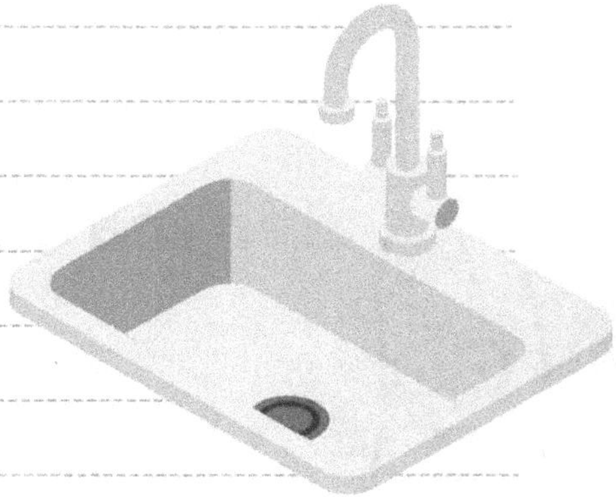

Potato Skins:

Citrus Peels:

Cucumber Peels:

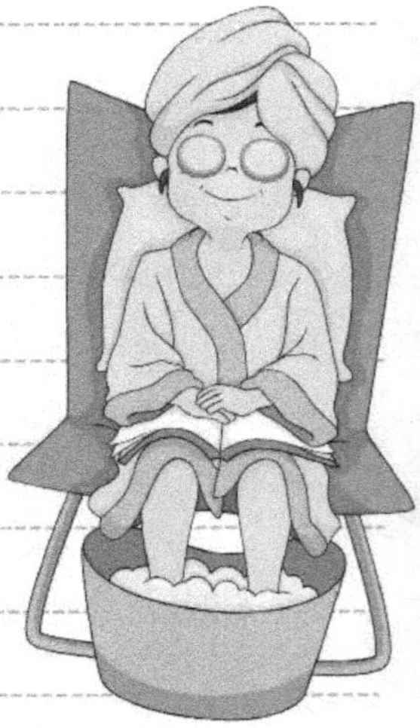

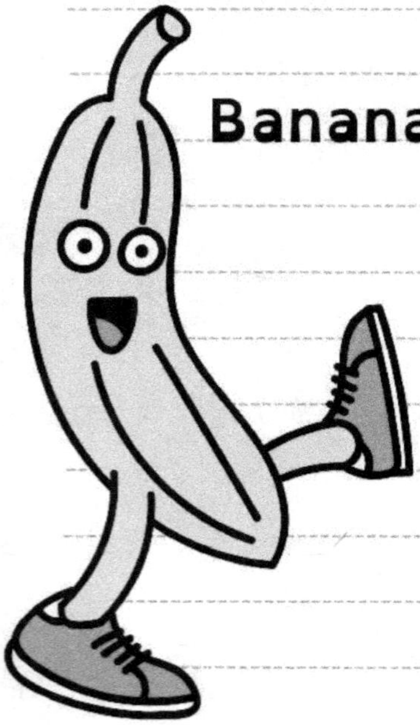

Banana Peels:

SWEET GREEN Smoothie

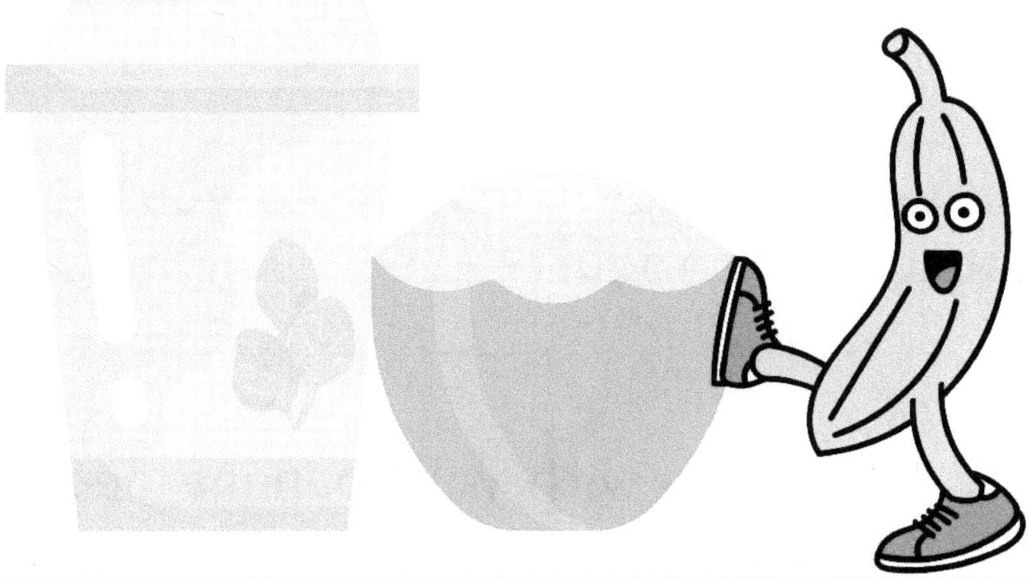

INGREDIENTS

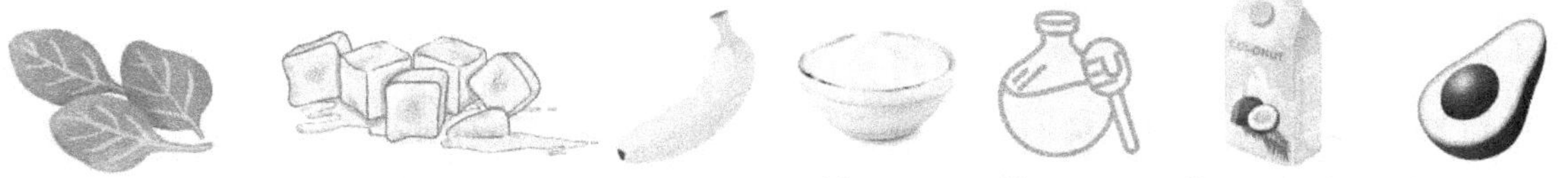

Spinach	Ice Cubes	Banana	Yogurt	Honey	Coconut Milk	Avocado

BLEND TOGETHER & ENJOY

1 cup Spinach 1/4 cup Ice Cubes 2 Bananas, peeled & frozen 1/4 cup Yogurt	2 Tablespoons Honey 2 cups Coconut Milk 1/2 Avocado, peeled & no seed *bonus* Splash of lemon juice

Smoothie Reflection Time

Did you enjoy this recipe?

Did you try the lemon juice?

Would you add anything more or less to this drink?

For a vegan recipe, what could you substitute for yogurt?

What did you do with your banana peel?

By naming a few health benefits this drink has, how could you describe, advertise, influence, or suggest this healthy drink to others?

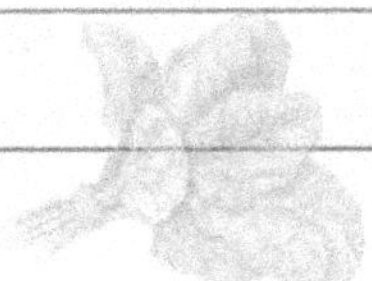

Rewrite your version of the recipe, making changes to quantities, steps, ingredients, or anything else you find fitting.

Recipe Name

Procedure

Yield

Cost

Time

Ingredients

How much would you charge for 16 oz?

What is your profit margin?

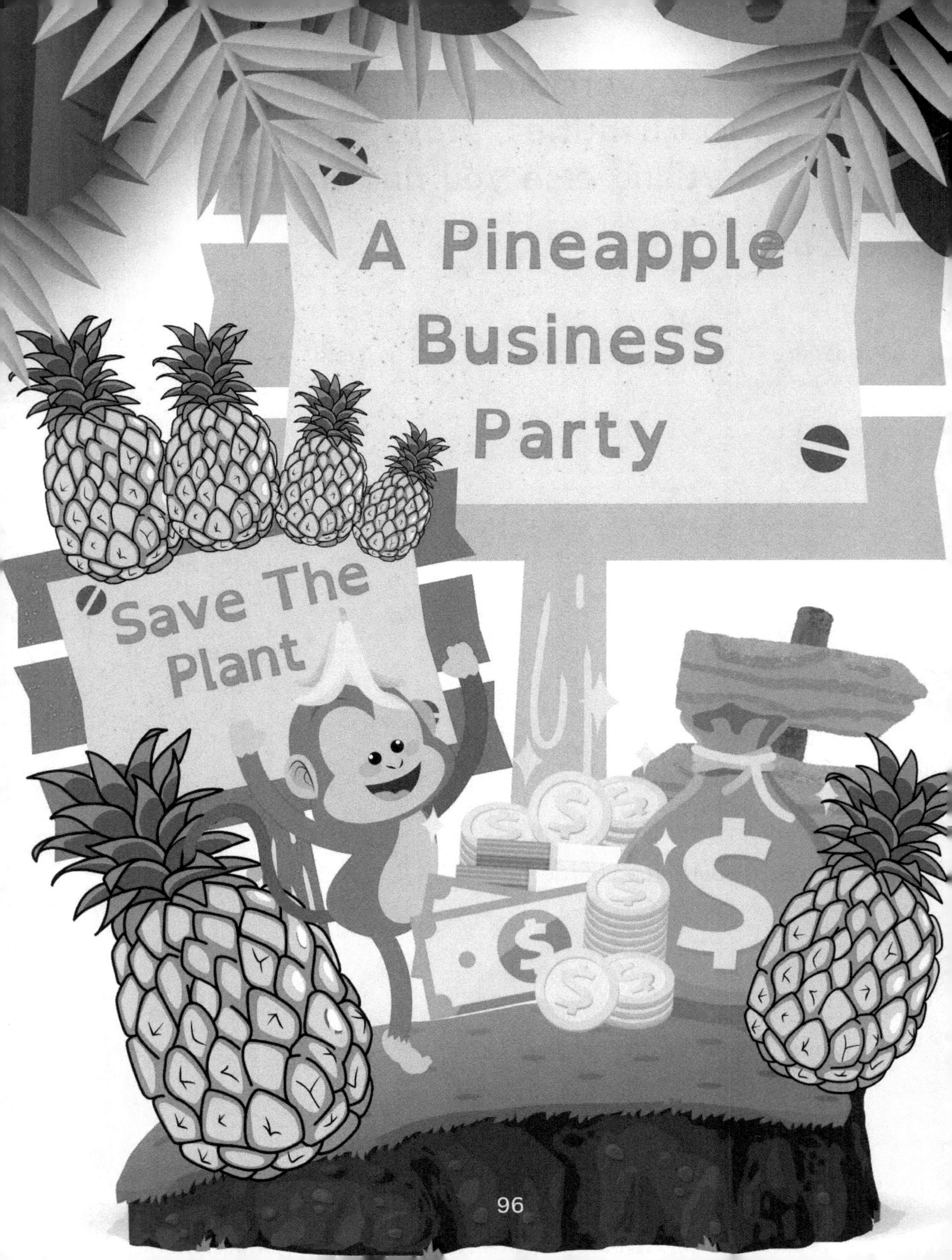
A Pineapple
Business
Party
Save The
Plant

Buy One, Grow One

Did you know you can grow pineapples? Pineapples are grown in the tropics and subtropics. What region do you live in? What fruits or vegetables can grow in your area?

How to plant:

- Cut the green top off, leaving about one inch of the fruit connected.
- Place the bottom of the green pineapple top in the dirt about 2-3 inches.
- Water and let grow. In about a year or two you will get another pineapple that will grow out of the center of the green top!
- Repeat.

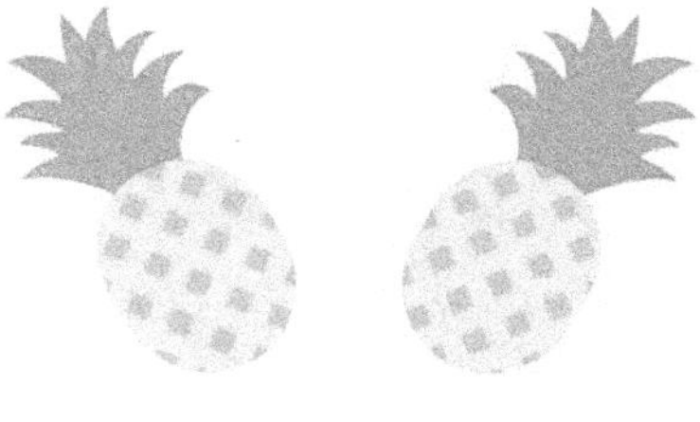

Pineapple Math

You decide to plant the pineapple you bought. Your garden now has 1 pineapple plant.

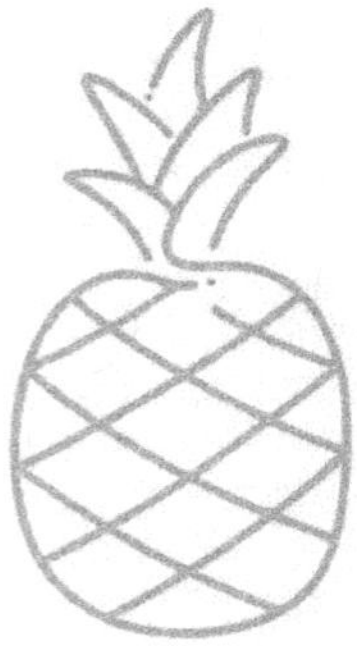

Year 1:
Your garden has produced 1 pineapple fruit. You decide top also plant the top from that pineapple fruit, now your garden has 2 pineapple plants.

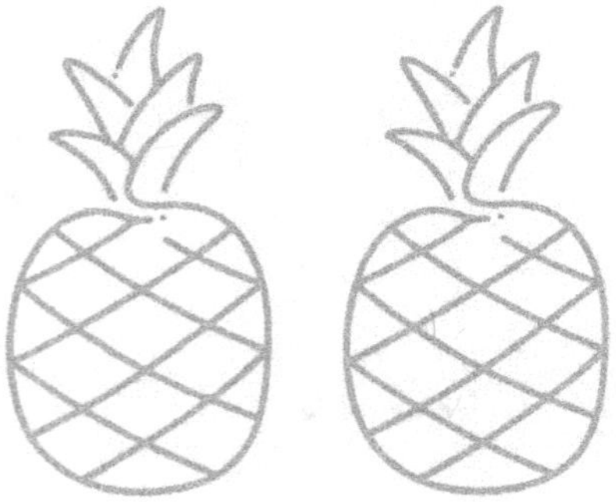

Year 2:
Your garden has produced 2 pineapple fruit. You plant these tops too, how many plants will be in your garden?

You decide you will continue to plant the pineapple tops from all of your pineapples. Answer the questions on the next page to find out how many pineapples you will have in the years to come.

Year 3:
Your garden has produced 4 pineapple fruit. How many plants will now be in your garden?

Year 4:
Your garden has ____ pineapple fruit. How many plants will now be in your garden?

Year 5:
Your garden has ____ pineapple fruit. How many plants will now be in your garden?

Year 6:
Your garden has ____ pineapple fruit. How many plants will now be in your garden?

Year 7:
Your garden has ____ pineapple fruit. How many plants will now be in your garden?

Running with Numbers

Your garden had **25** plants that all produced fruits **last year.** You sold your pineapples peeled, the green tops removed, and planted them in your garden. If each pineapple sells for $5, how much can you make **this year**?

If you started your own pineapple farm, by investing in 50 pineapple plants that were $10 each, how long would it take you to be able to pay off the investment by selling just the fruit at $5 each and planting the tops?

If you were to start your own pineapple fruit stand business, how many pineapple plants do you want to plant? Why?

How much will this cost, if each pineapple plant is $5?

What other business expenses would there be?

How much money could you make in the first 3 years?

How much space would you need for your garden? Draw the dimensions below of how much space one plant needs, then multiply this by the number of plants you want for your business. Use the space below to work out your answer.

If pineapples only fruit once, do you only get paid once a year? How do you financially plan for this?

What growing strategies could you do to ensure a healthy and reliable pineapple fruit production each year?

Where would you sell your pineapples?

How would you advertise?

Is this a business you want to start?

What other business or businesses would you want to make?

TROPICAL Smoothie

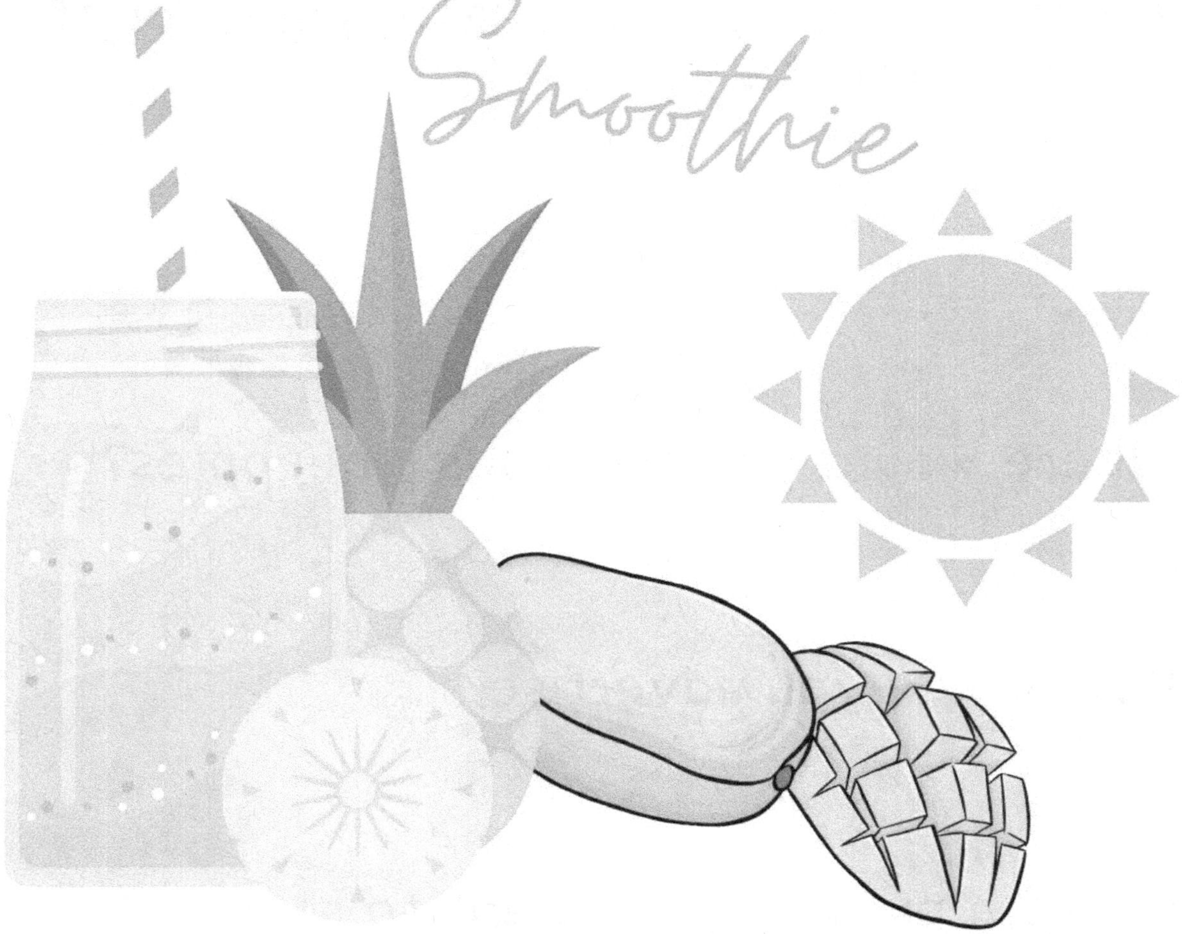

INGREDIENTS

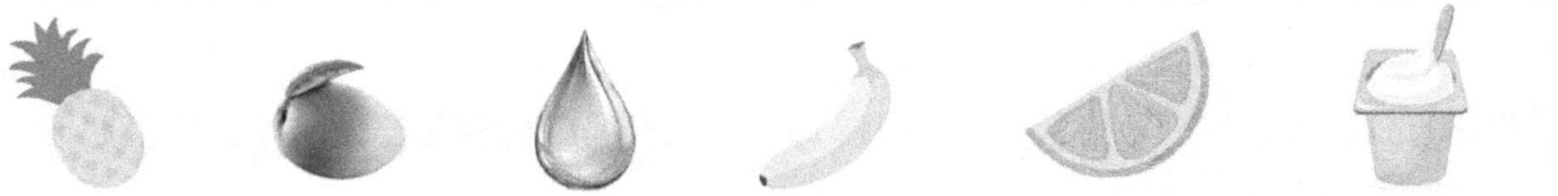

Pineapple	Mango	Water	Banana	OrangeJuice	Greek Yogurt

BLEND TOGETHER & ENJOY

1/2 cup Pineapple Chunks 1/2 cup Mango Chunks 1 cup Water	1 Banana, peeled & frozen 1 cup Orange Juice 1/2 cup Greek Yogurt

Smoothie Reflection Time

Did you like this recipe and smoothie?

Would you make any changes to the ingredient list? Like using different liquids?

Was it sweet, tangy, sour, spicy or tart? Use descriptive words to tell someone about this smoothie.

By naming a few health benefits this drink has, how could you describe, advertise, influence, or suggest this healthy drink to others?

How much money would you pay for this smoothie if you were at a cafe?

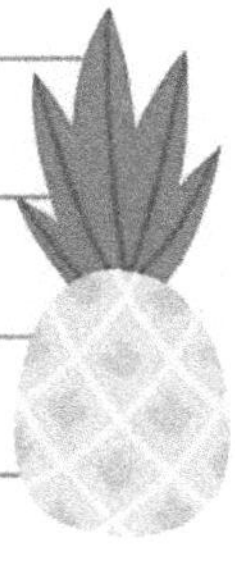

Rewrite your version of the recipe, making changes to quantities, steps, ingredients, or anything else you find fitting.

Recipe Name

Procedure

Yield

Cost

Time

Ingredients

How much would you charge for 16 oz?

What is your profit margin?

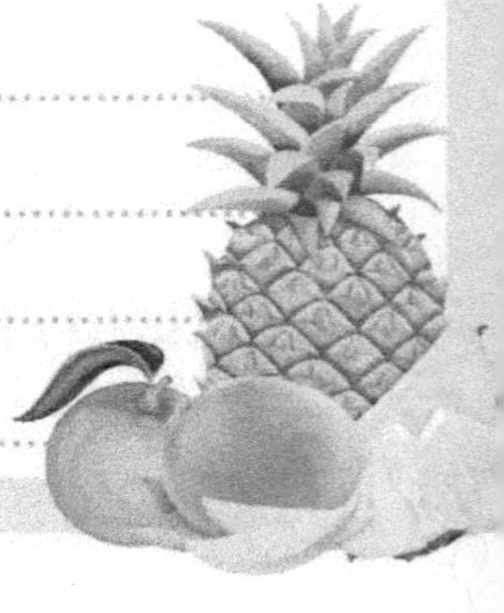

Got Grain on the Brain?

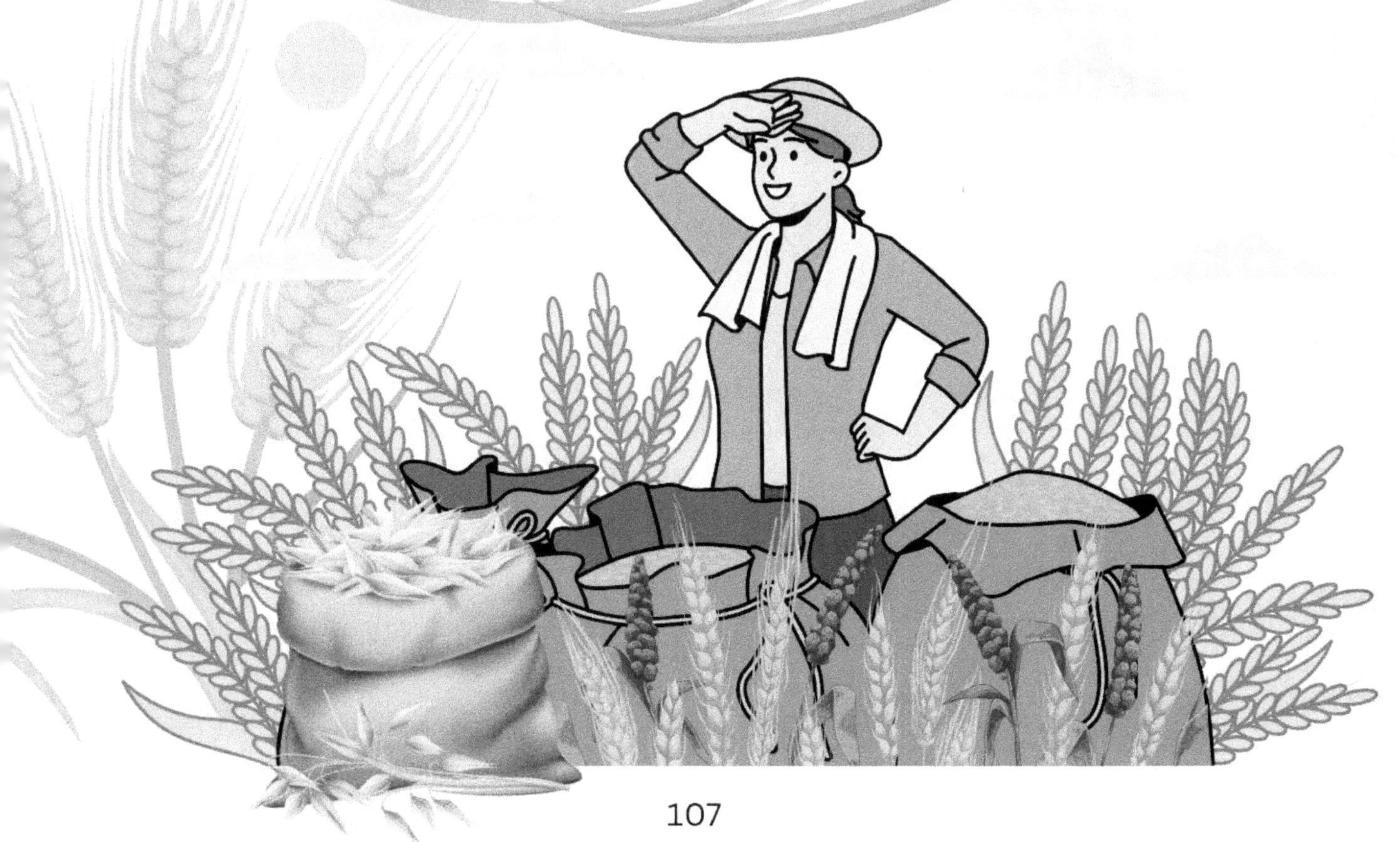

Grain Search

I	Y	A	L	W	W	O	B	S	C	R	G	C	X	S
I	L	P	H	P	F	A	A	M	P	O	Y	B	A	P
V	A	E	C	Y	H	L	R	K	X	S	U	E	O	E
A	A	A	H	O	Q	N	L	X	Z	C	U	V	N	L
T	H	X	K	X	R	L	E	P	K	P	R	K	I	T
M	B	J	F	A	S	N	Y	W	D	B	A	Y	U	E
M	I	L	L	E	T	T	H	Y	M	M	Q	J	Q	S
G	Y	R	E	Q	L	E	A	X	E	F	X	I	L	Z
F	T	C	I	B	A	X	W	O	I	D	V	E	Y	S
A	I	J	S	T	T	M	D	D	N	S	Y	F	M	M
R	I	L	S	N	P	M	S	Q	P	N	J	B	V	I
C	S	O	E	O	R	E	C	I	R	D	L	I	W	X
C	U	R	M	E	H	C	W	O	N	L	V	W	O	S
A	U	H	H	R	E	G	L	U	B	W	X	F	Q	R
F	R	Q	B	A	Z	Y	U	C	K	S	O	A	S	M

Corn	Barley	Buckwheat
Bulger	Oats	Quinoa
Rice	Millet	Rye
Spelt	Wheat	Wild Rice

There are over 20 grain varieties. Find what they are, write them down, describe the health aspects of each, where they are grown, and if these grains are available in your local food markets.

Practice your cursive handwriting skills!

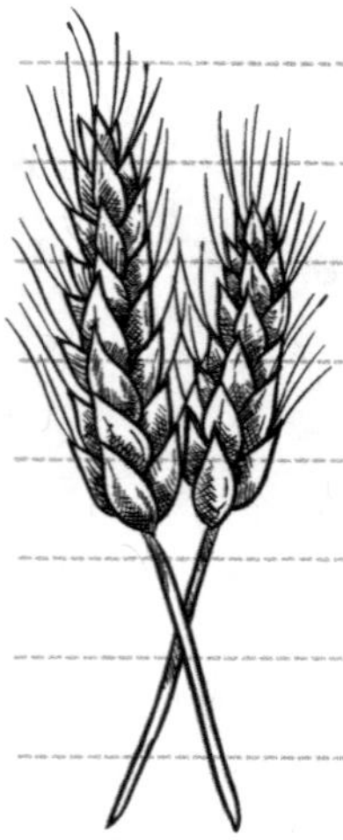

Grainy Breakdown

Use this space to draw and label the three parts of a whole grain: Bran, Germ, and Endosperm.

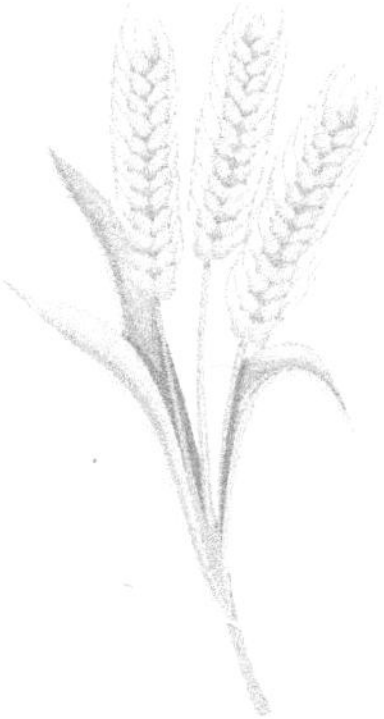

Explain where most of the fiber and nutrients come from in the grain: bran, germ, or endosperm.

What is the difference between a whole grain and a refined grain?

Are most packaged flours that are purchased in a store whole or refined grain? Explain.

What types of foods use refined grains and not whole grains in their recipes? Why?

Should these types of foods be consumed several times a day? Explain.

Research and explain how these foods effect our mood.

List the similarities and differences.

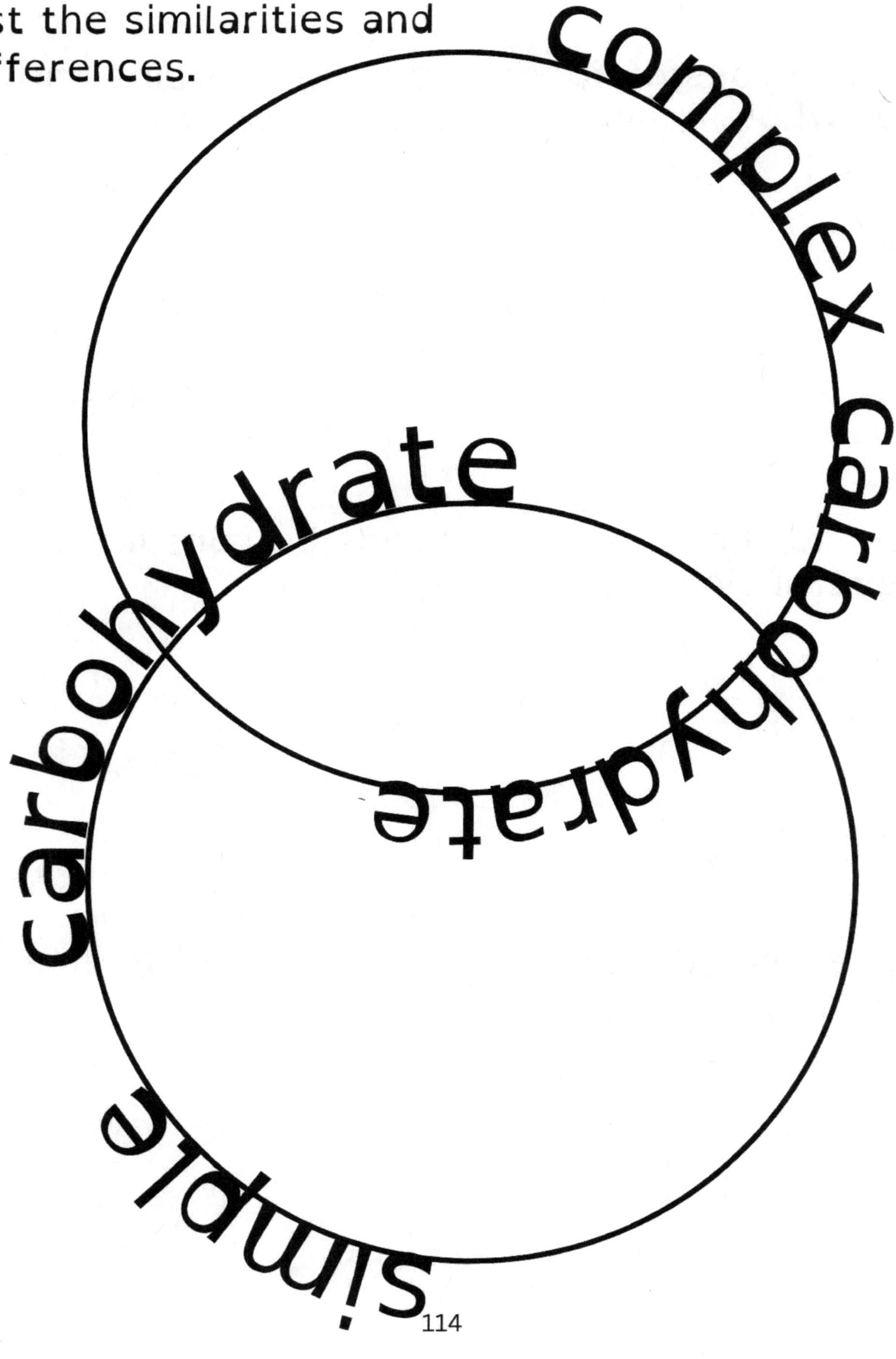

Bread Dough

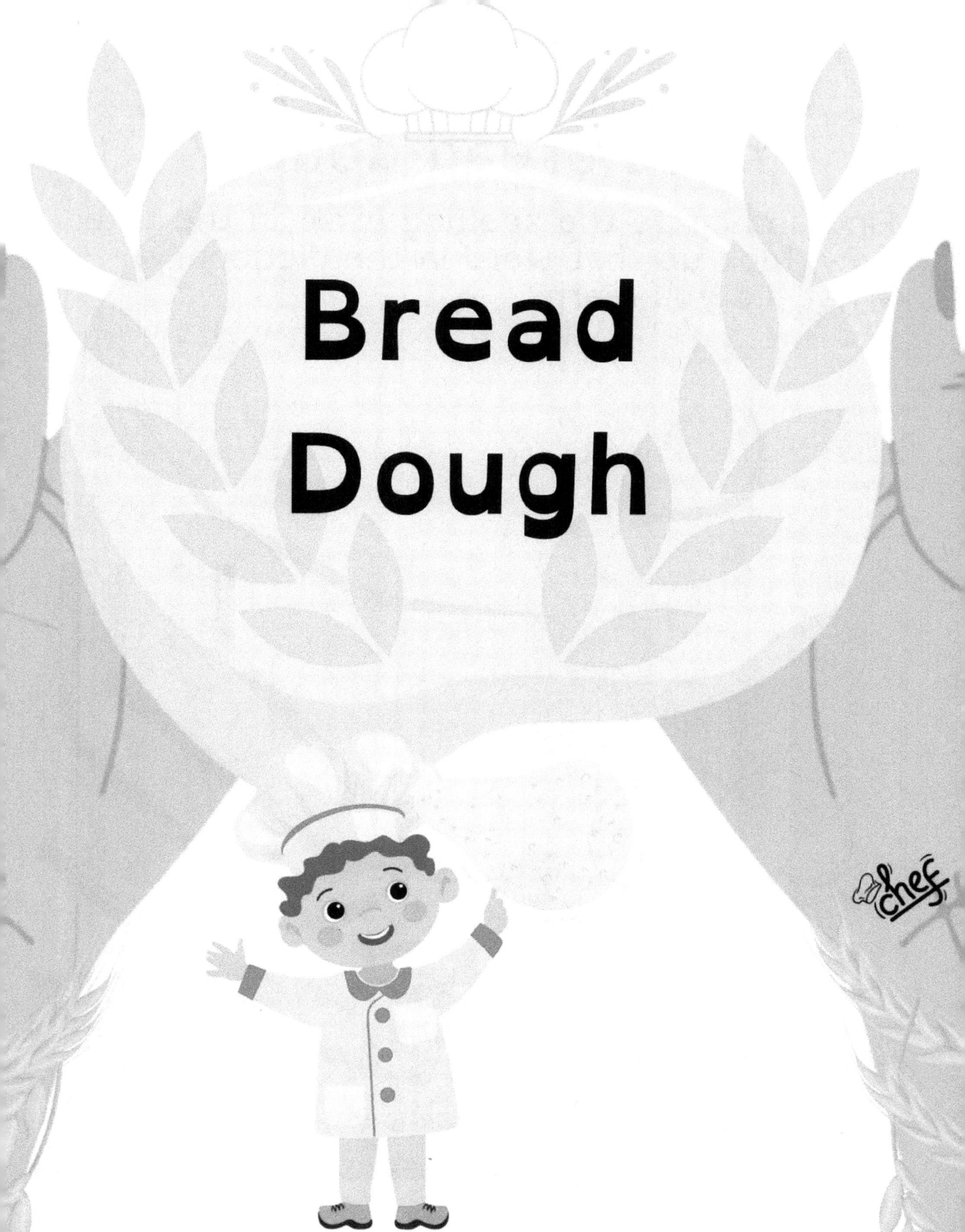

What do you knead to make bread dough?

Find and circle the spelling error in the title.
Now, look up that word in the dictionary.
What did you learn?

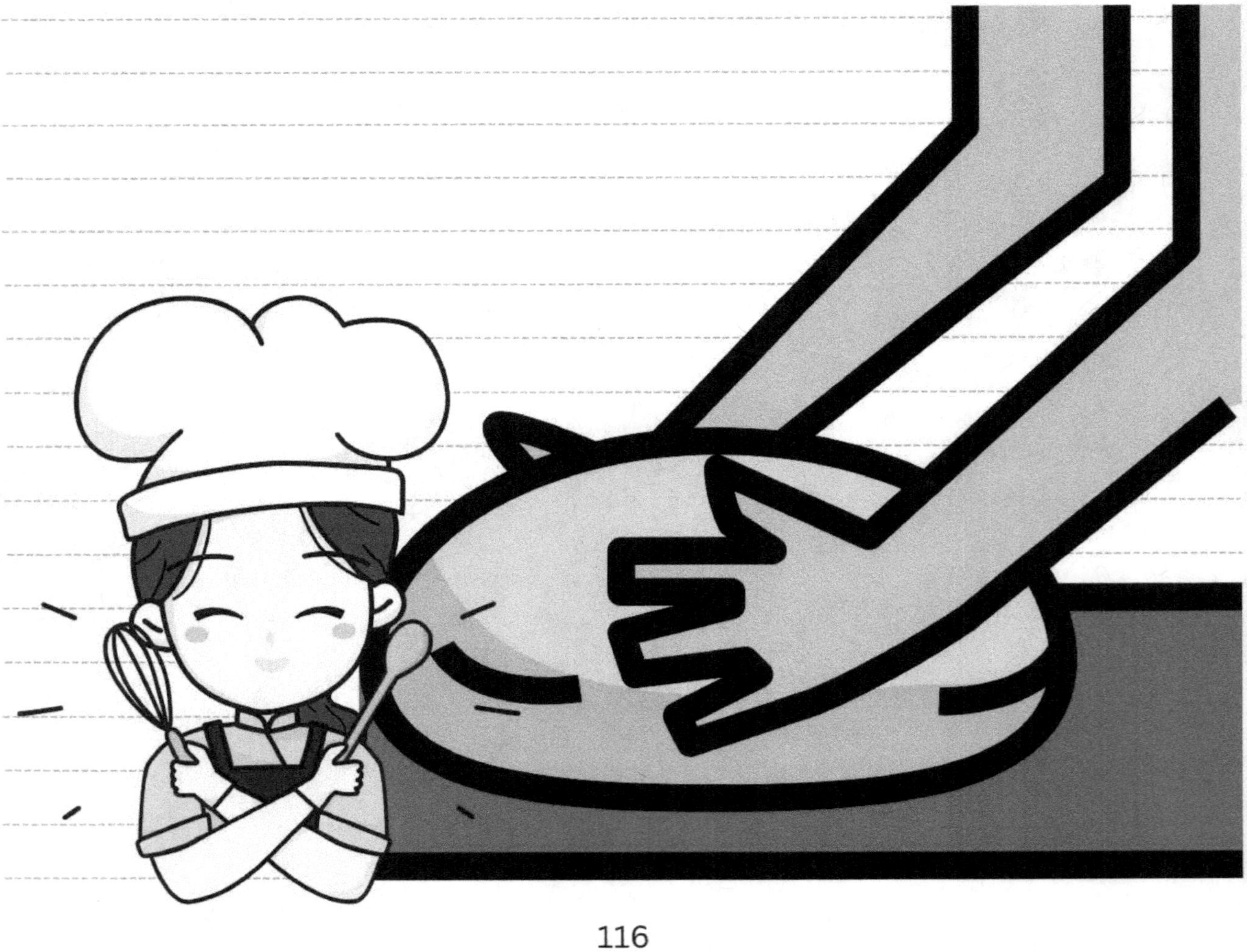

1. Make the dough...

...What ingredients and supplies do you need to make bread? Research, describe, and label.

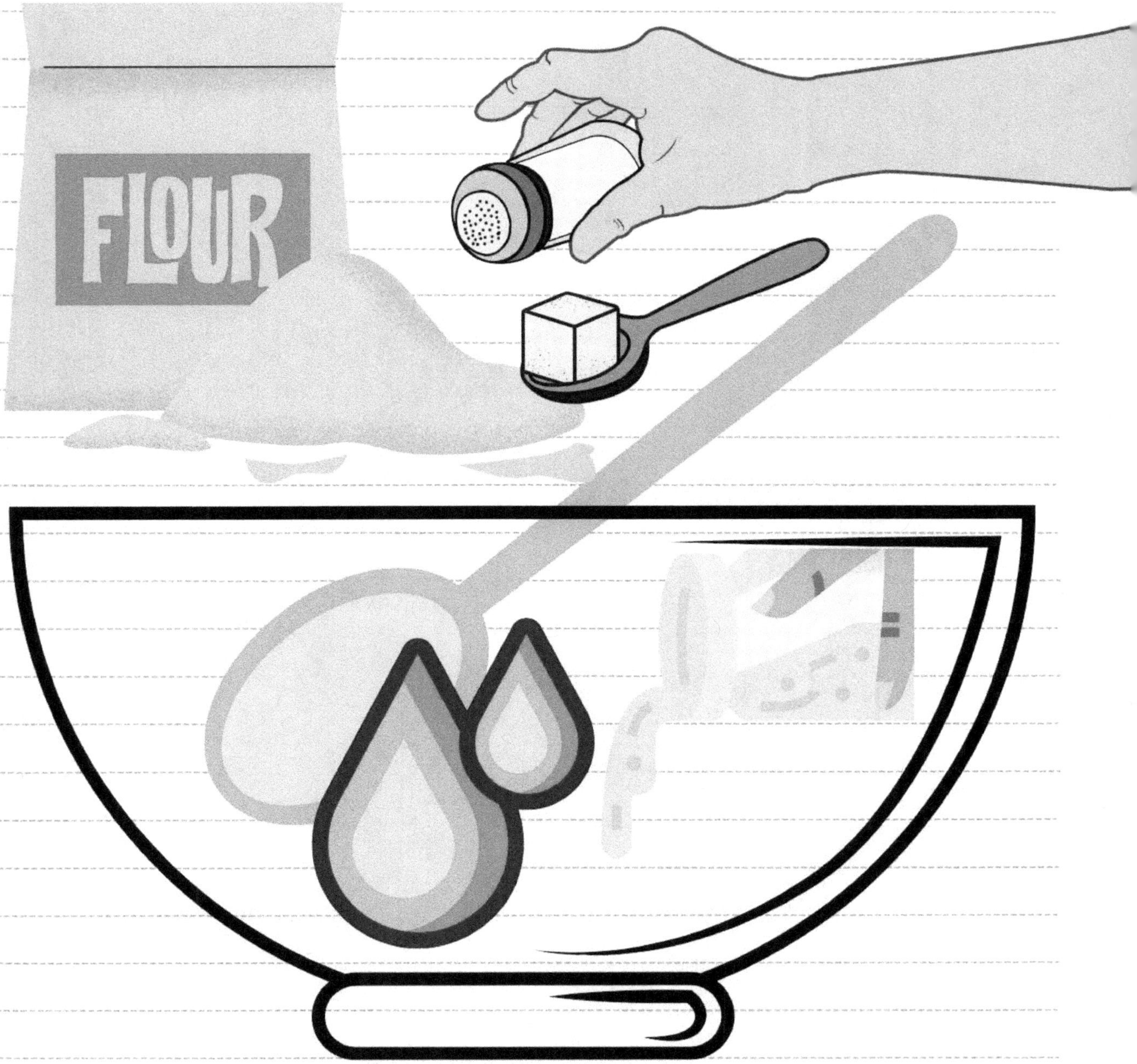

2. Knead the dough...

Research, describe, and label.

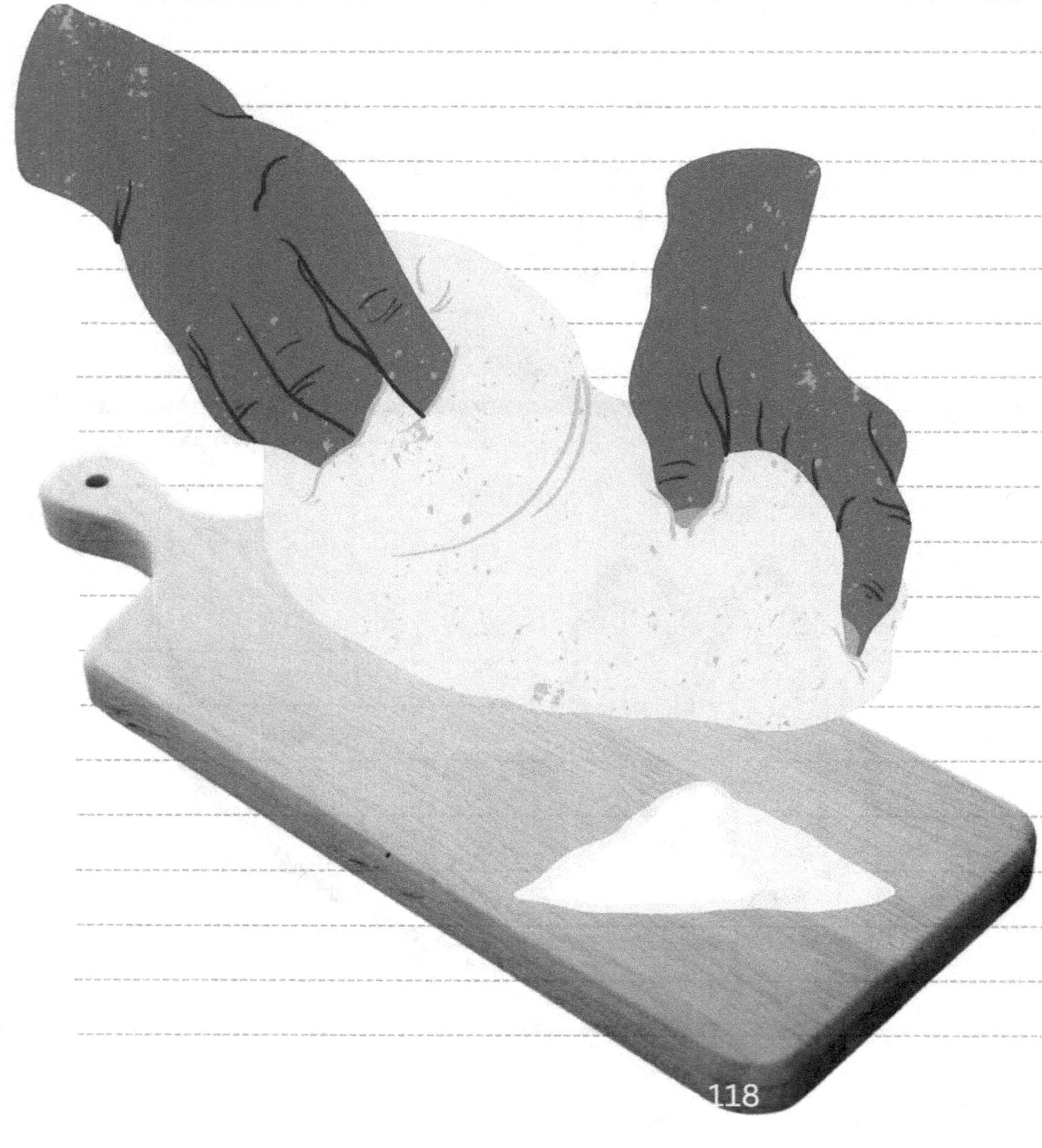

3. Let the dough rise

Research, describe, and label.

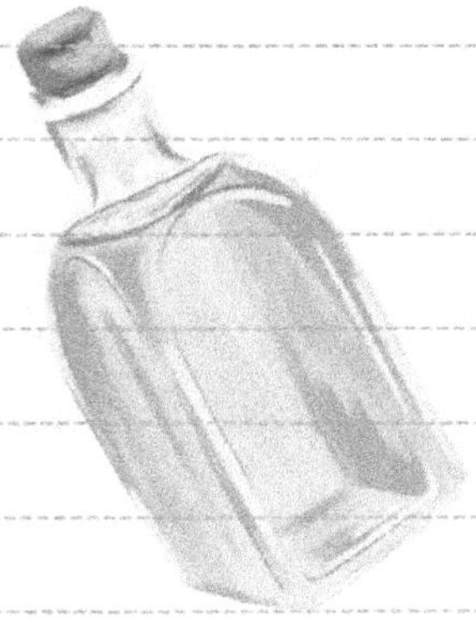

4. Bake the dough

Research, describe, and label.

5. Cool off and enjoy!

Now find a bread recipe you want to make!
Write about your experience.

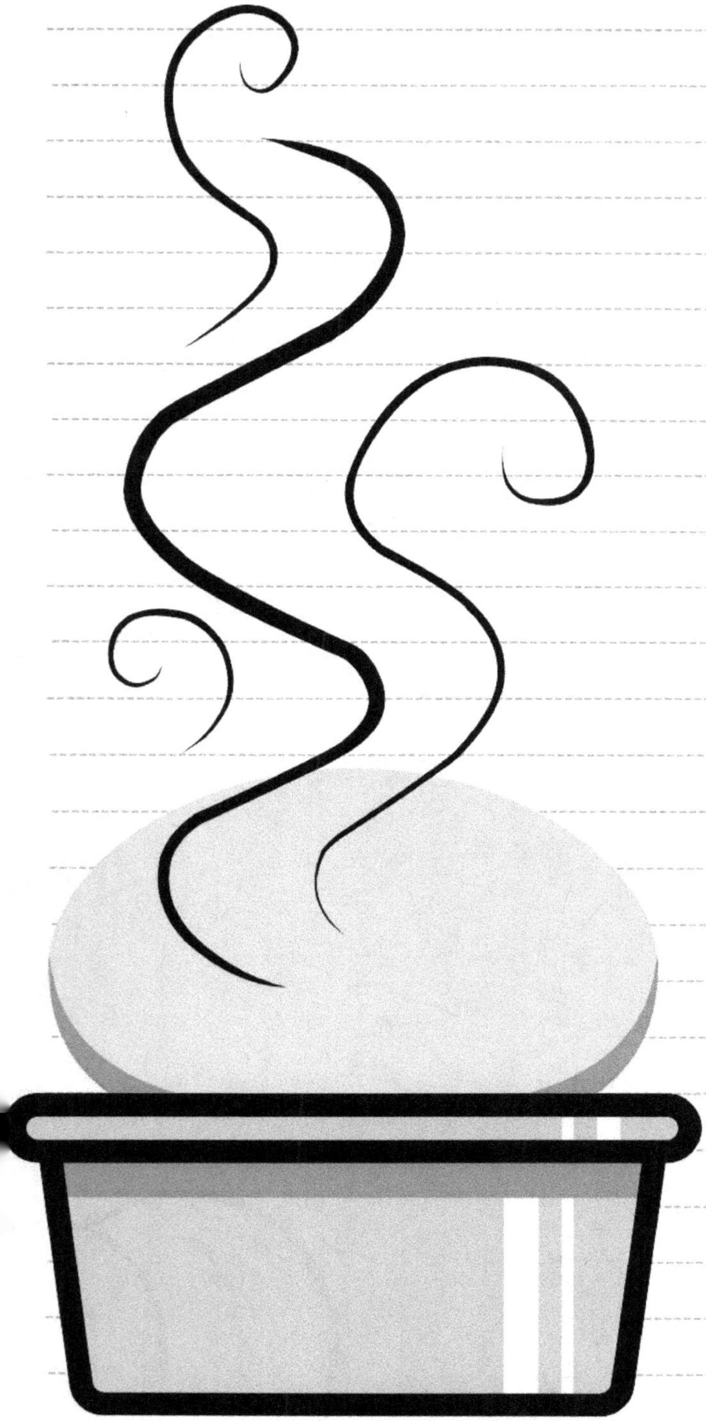

A Delicious Bread Recipe

Ingredients

______________________ ______________________

______________________ ______________________

______________________ ______________________

______________________ ______________________

Yield: Prep Time: Cook Time:

Directions

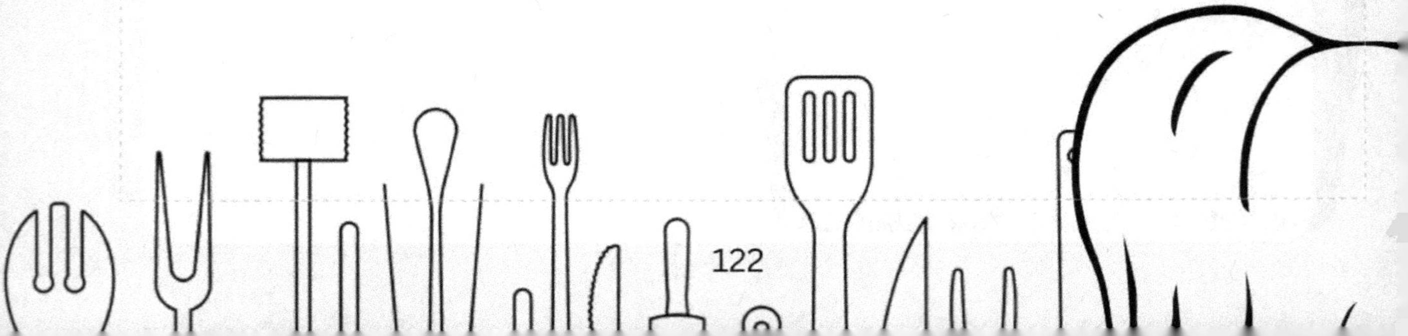

Grainy Math

Bread Recipe Conversion

A bread recipe calls for:
2 parts flour
1 part water

How much water would you need if you were to use 4 cups of flour?
_________ cups of water.

Fill in the blanks on the rest of the conversion problems.

_________ cups of flour
___1/4___ cups of water

Now double that...

_________ cups of flour
_________ cups of water

Now double that once more...

_________ cups of flour
_________ cups of water

Hint: You should have wound up with the answer from the first question.

ANSWER: 4 cups flour & 1 cup water

Continue and double again.

_________ cups of flour
_________ cups of water

double again...

_________ cups of flour
_________ cups of water

Now reduce the recipe by cutting your previous measurements in half...

_________ cups of flour
_________ cups of water

Reduce the quantities 50%...

_________ cups of flour
_________ cups of water

and another 50%...

_________ cups of flour
_________ cups of water

and another 50%...

_________ cups of flour
_________ cups of water

The Flour Journey

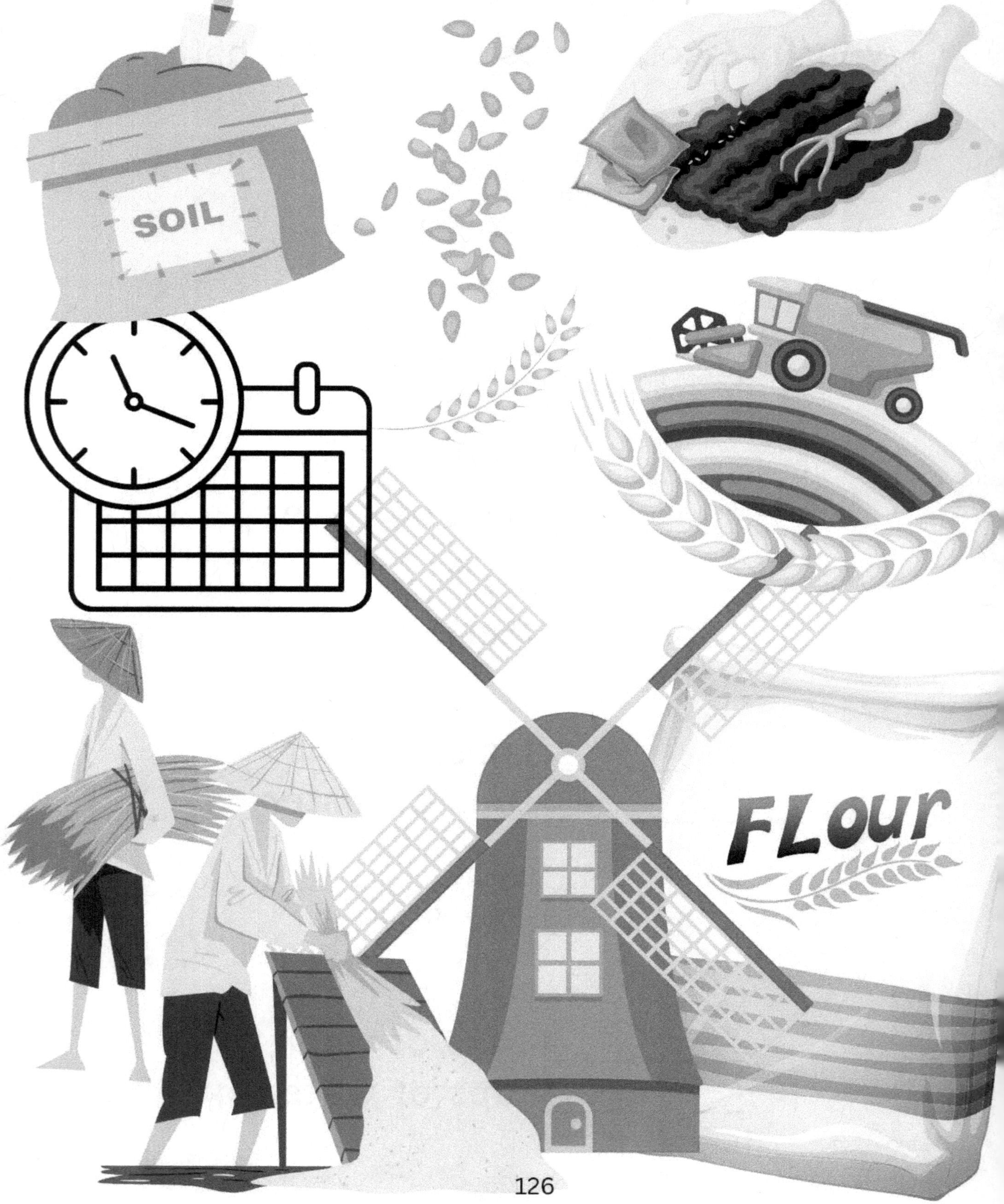

Explain the process from seed to flour. Use the pictures for help, but get more details in your research. For example, describe how long wheat takes from seed to harvest.

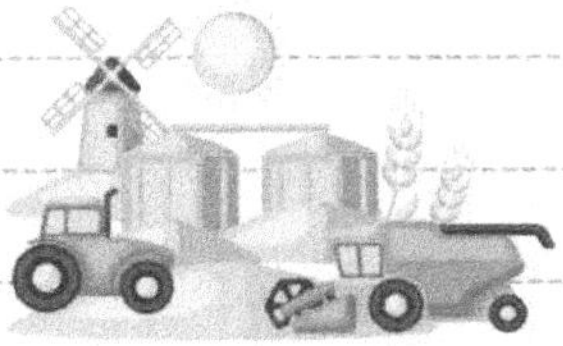

Name the many different types of flour you find in your research and briefly describe their unique nutritional qualities. Do you find these flours in your local market?

Practice your cursive handwriting skills!

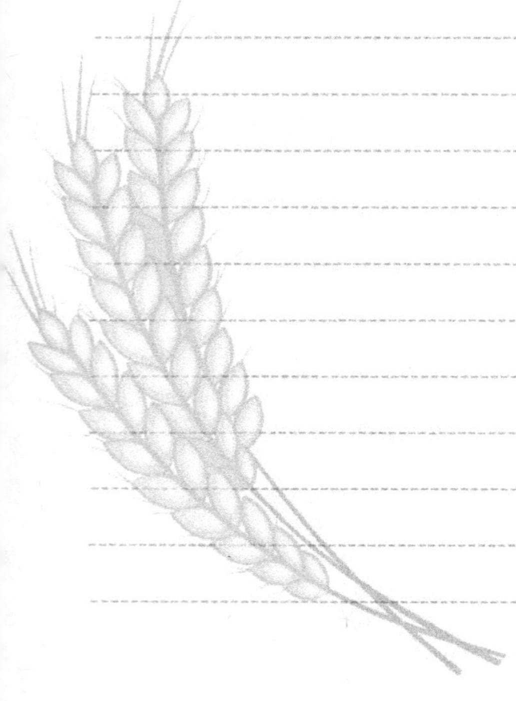

What is yeast?

What are the different types of yeast used for in baking?

Can there be yeast alternatives in baking?

What are Nutritional Yeast Flakes and is this similar to the yeast used in bread making? Explain.

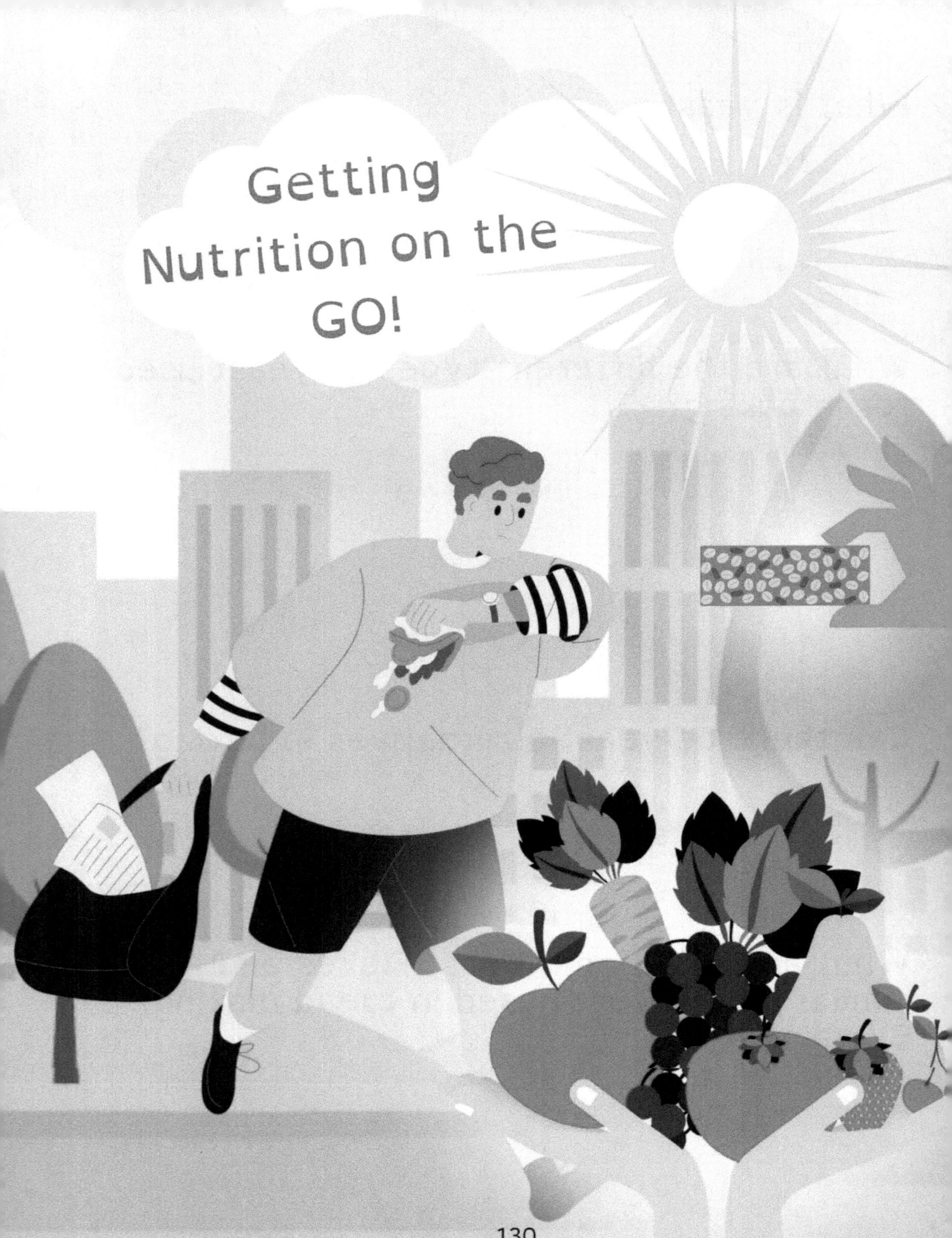
Getting
Nutrition on the
GO!

Ingredients Packed Full of Nutrients

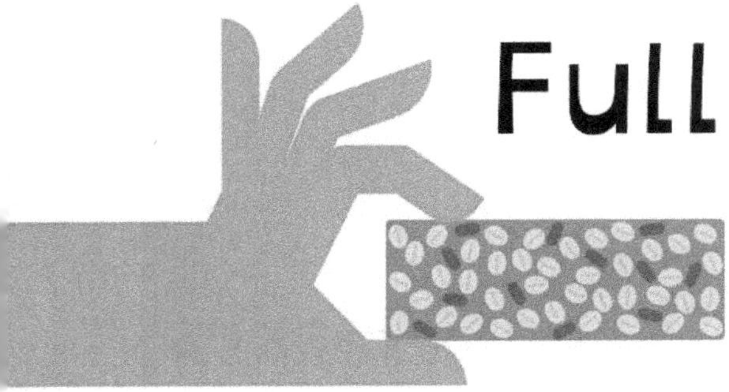

Granola or trail mix can be a hidden gem of nutrient dense ingredients, yet so tasty and simple to eat on the go! Below are just a few great ingredients you can add to your mixes. Beside each food name, describe at least one health quality the food contains.

Cashews

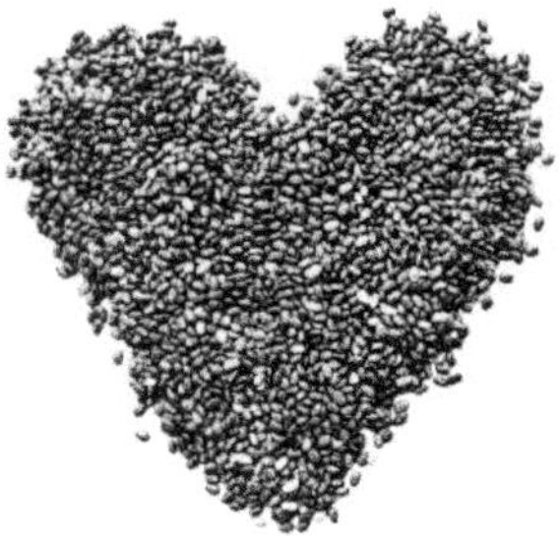

Honey

Chia Seeds

Dried Cranberries

Pumpkin Seeds

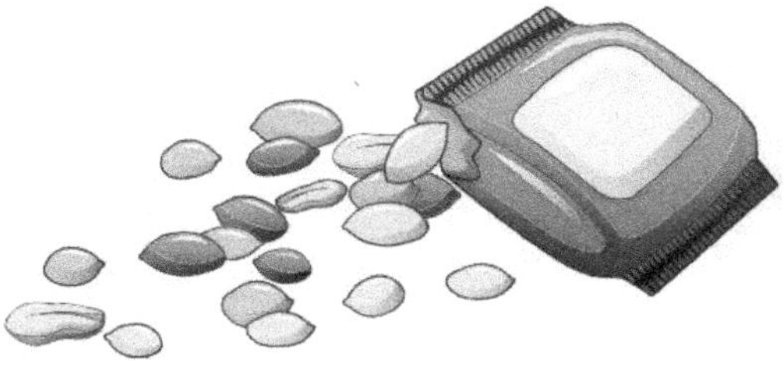

Bee Pollen

Cacao Nibs

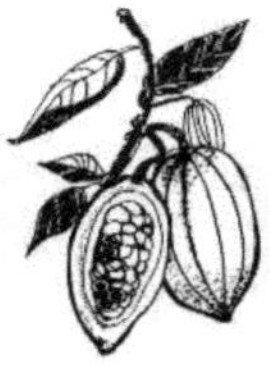

Raisins

Coconut Flakes

Dried Tart Cherries

MCT Oil

Gogi Berries

Almond Butter

Nutritional Yeast Flakes

Oatmeal

Monk Fruit

Black Strap Molasses

Granola Fun Recipe

Find and write out a granola recipe, make any changes that work best for you.

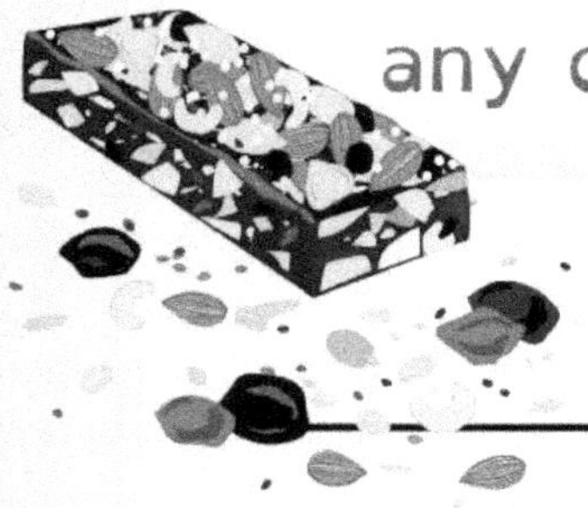

Ingredients

Yield: Prep Time: Cook Time:

Directions

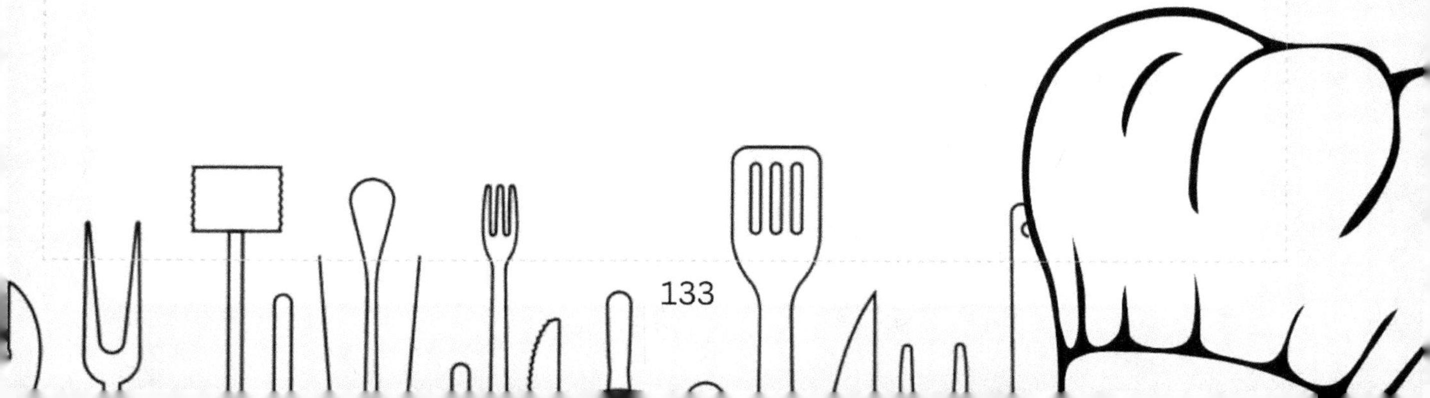

Granola Reflection Time

Did you expect this recipe to taste the way it did?

Would you want to make different variations of this recipe, for example a coconut and pineapple batch or a chocolate and peanut butter mix? Name a few other variations you can think of.

What additional healthy foods would you want to add to your granola?

Could you sell this at a local market? How much would you sell it for? Explain.

Fun Foods

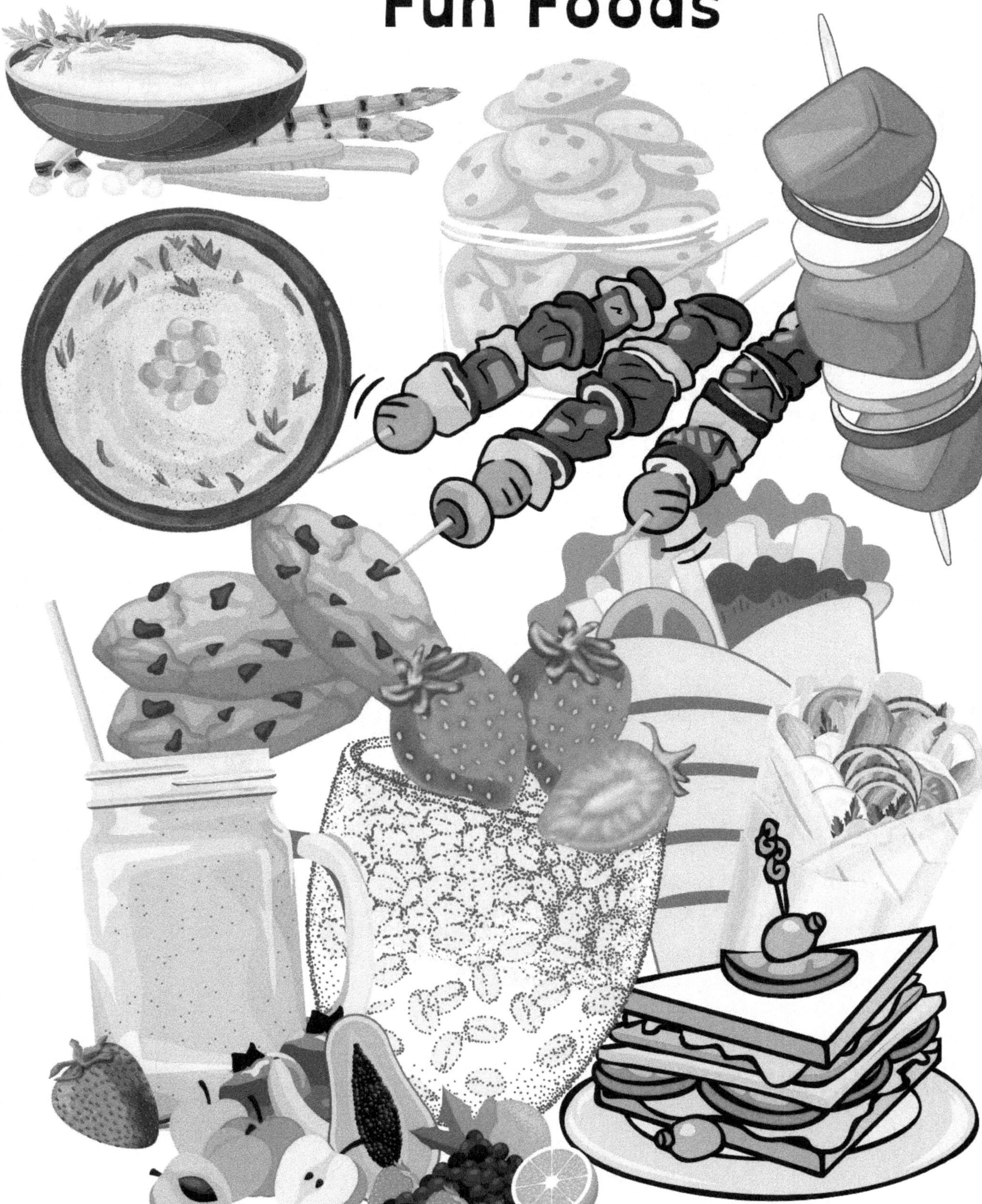

With a few more nutrition on the go ideas, describe some healthy ingredients to use when making each healthy snack or meal.

Sandwiches:

Healthy Cookies:

Smoothies:

Yogurt Parfait:

Kabobs:

Wraps:

Hummus:

Salad/Fruit Salad:

Fun Foods

List fun ways to combine and eat these foods.

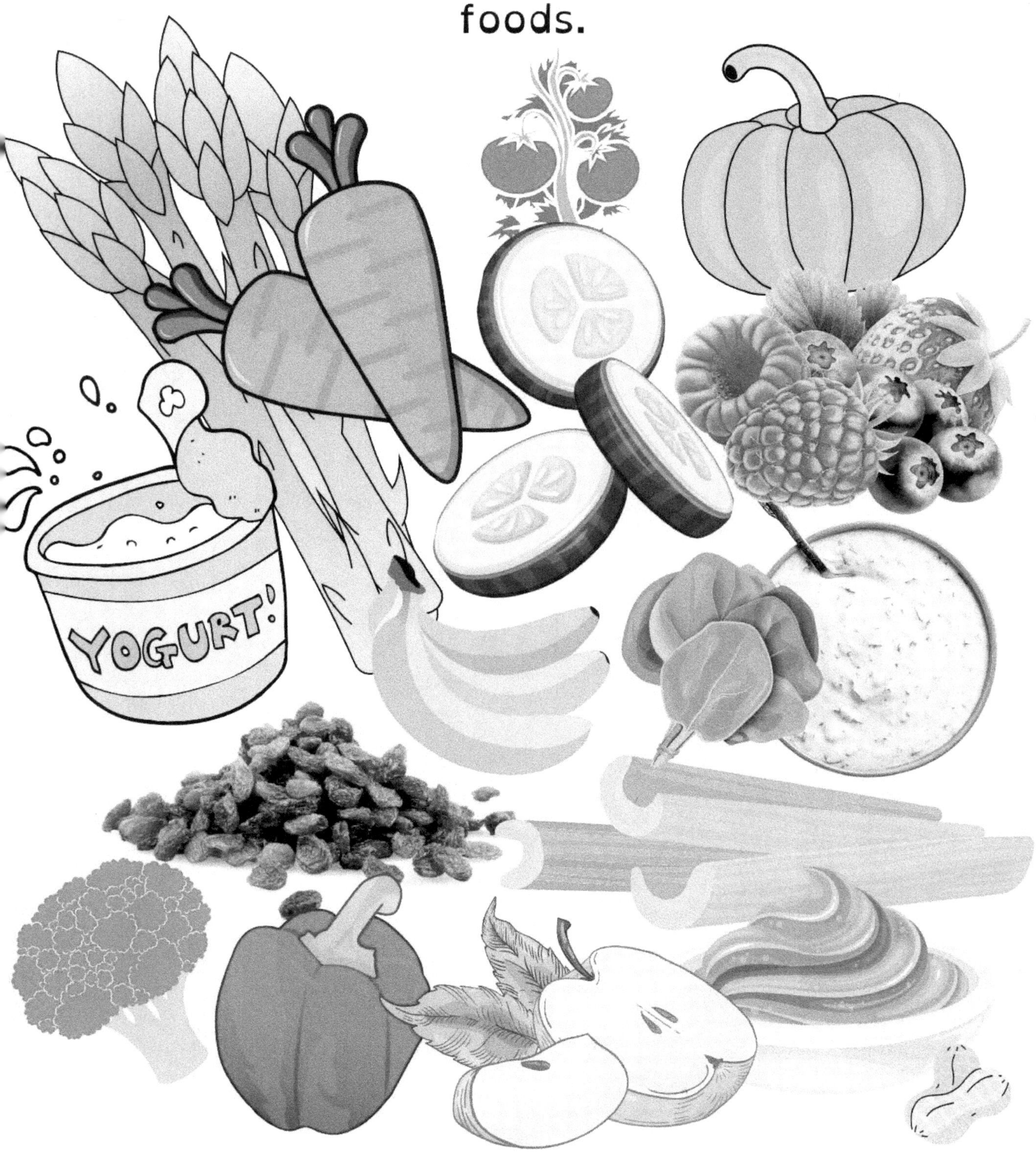

Practice your cursive handwriting skills!

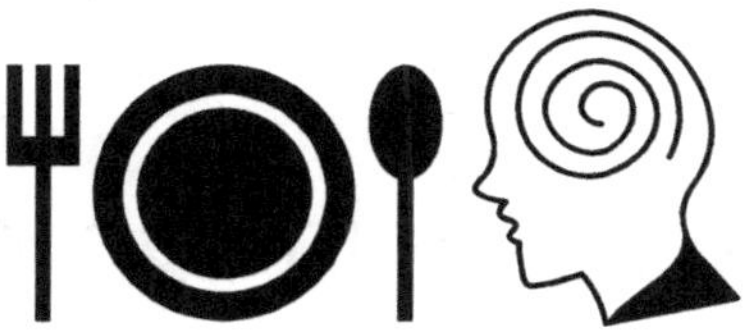

Mindful Eating

Eating does not have to be rushed, even if it is on the go. Research and describe what mindful eating is, the benefits, and a few mindful eating tips and techniques you can do.

Describe the way you normally eat your food. Can you improve this with mindful eating techniques?

Do you eat with thought and appreciation of the food and preparation?

Do you say thanks or pray before or during your meal? Explain.

Reflect and apply some mindful eating and even food making habits that can be beneficial to your mind, body, mood, and energy.

Kitchen Conversions

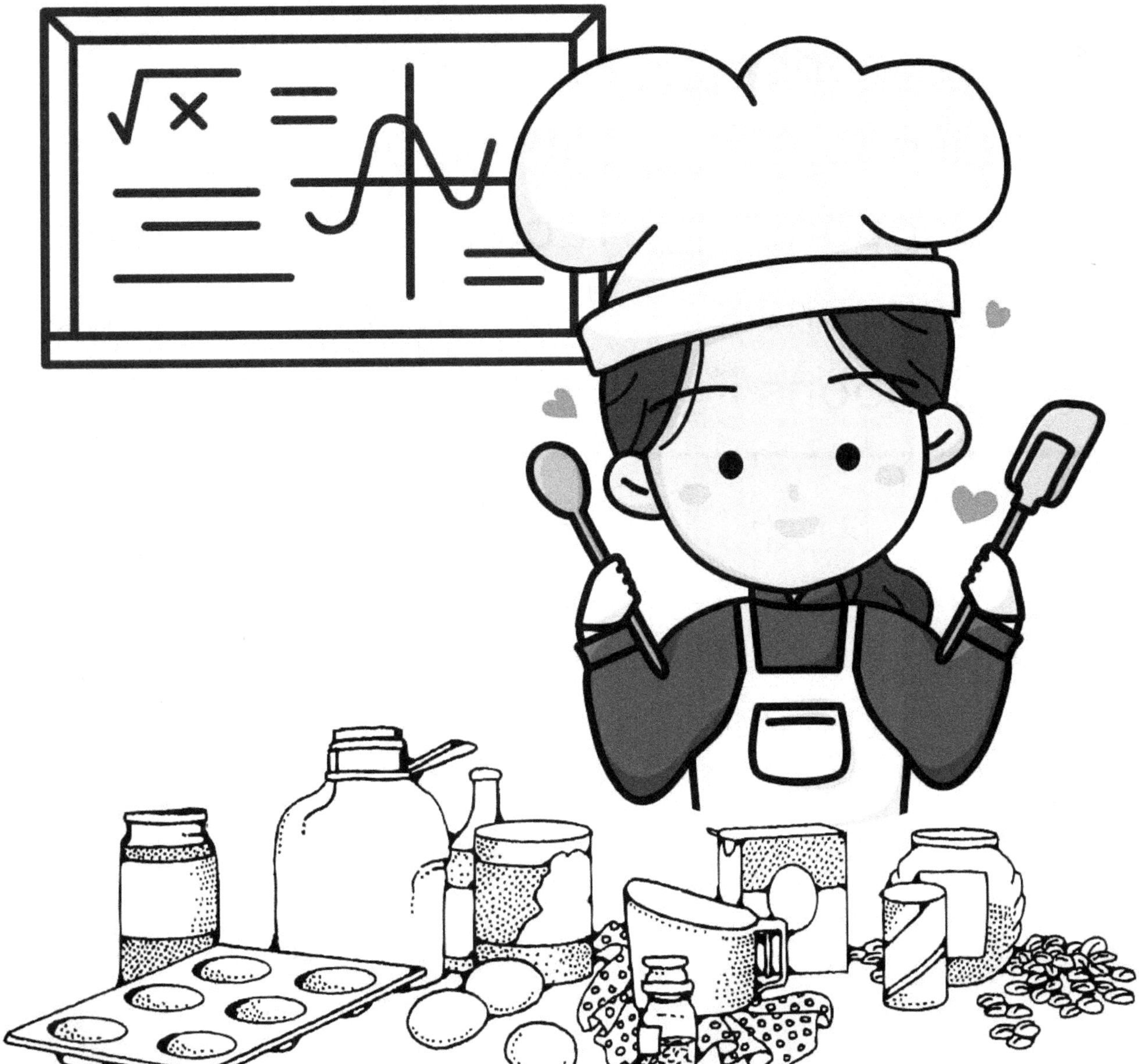

Dry Ingredients

Fill in the blanks by using the first line as a clue to answer the next blanks. Use the space below for your calculations.

3 teaspoons = 1 Tablespoon = 1/16 cup

6 teaspoons = ___ Tablespoons = ___ cup

12 teaspoons = ___ Tablespoons = ___ cup

24 teaspoons = ___ Tablespoons = ___ cup

36 teaspoons = ___ Tablespoons = ___ cup

48 teaspoons = ___ Tablespoons = ___ cup

Circle the examples of dry ingredients.

Yogurt

Wheat Bran

Almond Flour

Milk

Sugar

Flour

Brown Sugar

Oatmeal

Butter

Chocolate Chips

Flaxseed

Honey

Cocoa Powder

Wet Ingredients

Fill in the blanks by using the first line as a clue to answer the next blanks. Use the space below for your calculations.

4 ounces=	1/2 cup =	1/4 pint =	1/8 quart
8 ounces=	___ cup =	___ pint =	___ quart
12 ounces=	___ cup =	___ pint =	___ quart
16 ounces=	___ cup =	___ pint =	___ quart
32 ounces=	___ cup =	___ pint =	___ quart
___ ounces=	___ cup =	___ pint =	1 gallon

How many quarts make up a gallon?

Circle the examples of wet ingredients.

Kefir

Juice

Chia Seeds

Cream Cheese

Pistachios

Cashew Milk

Molasses

Quinoa

Water

Maple Syrup

Rice

Bee Pollen

Agave Syrup

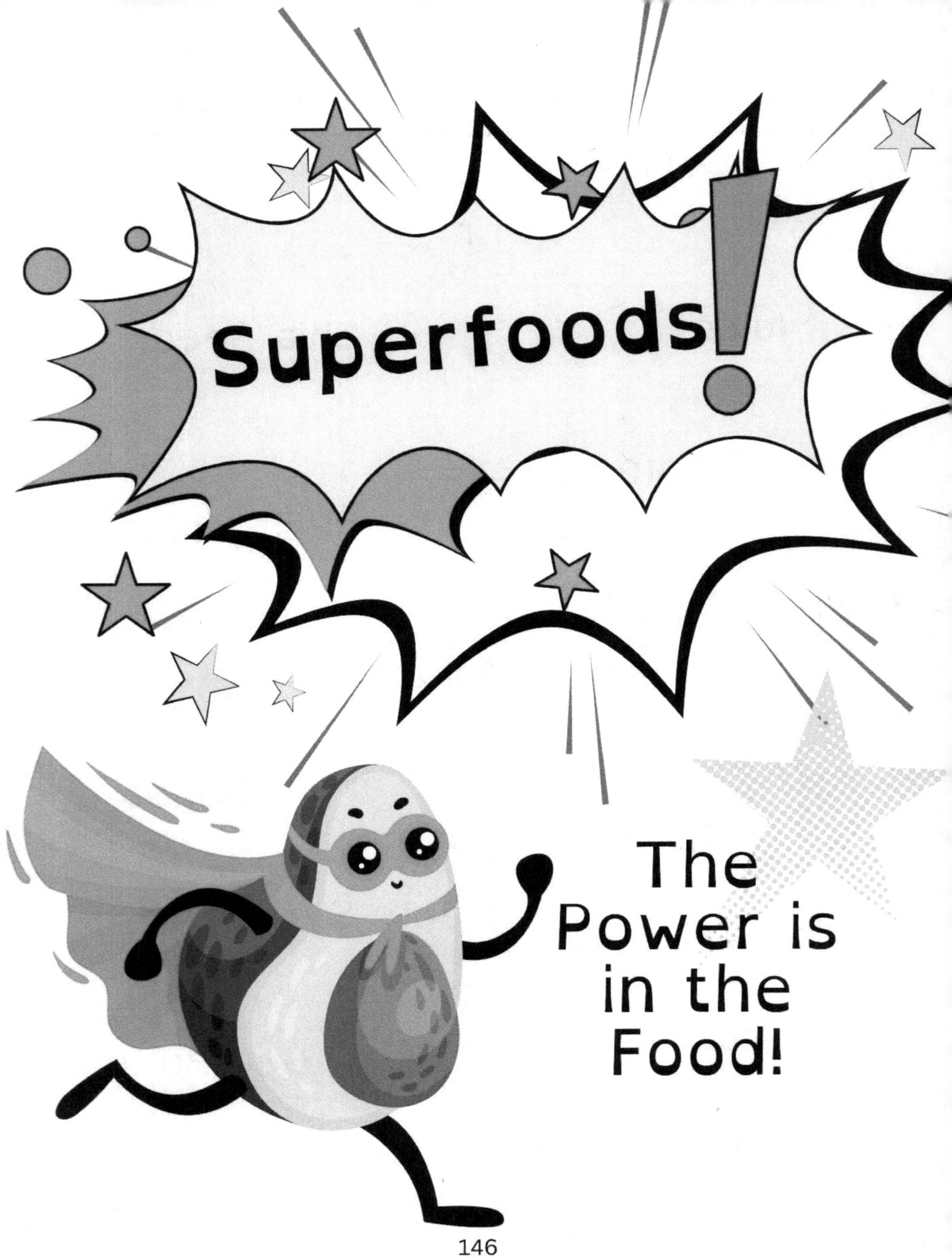
Superfoods!
The Power is in the Food!

Superfoods

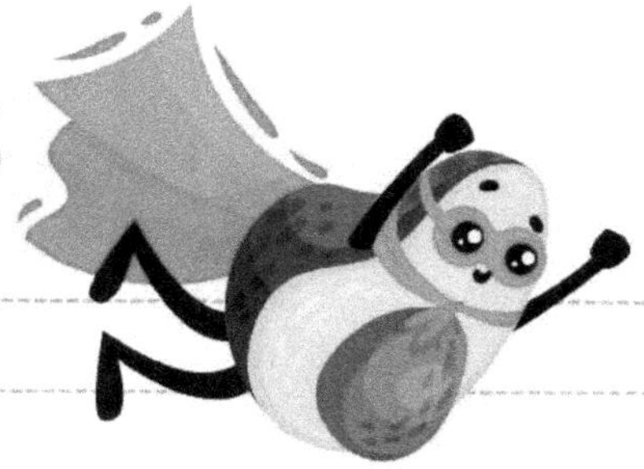

What classifies a superfood?

How often do you eat superfoods?

How can you incorporate more into your diet?

Do you need to be cautious of pesticides even if a food is a superfood?

Can you tell a difference in energy level or mood after eating superfoods?

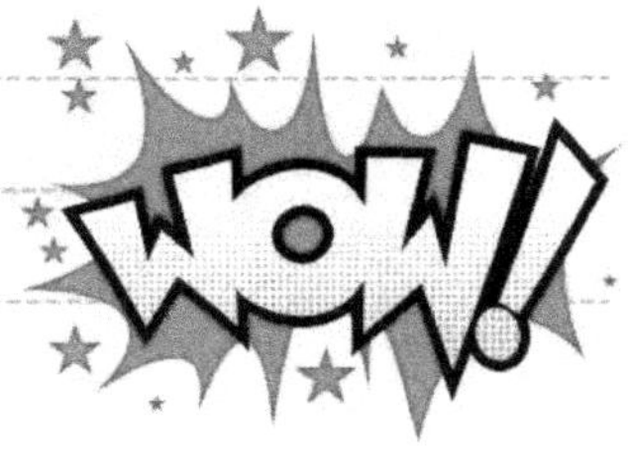

Circle and label the superfoods.

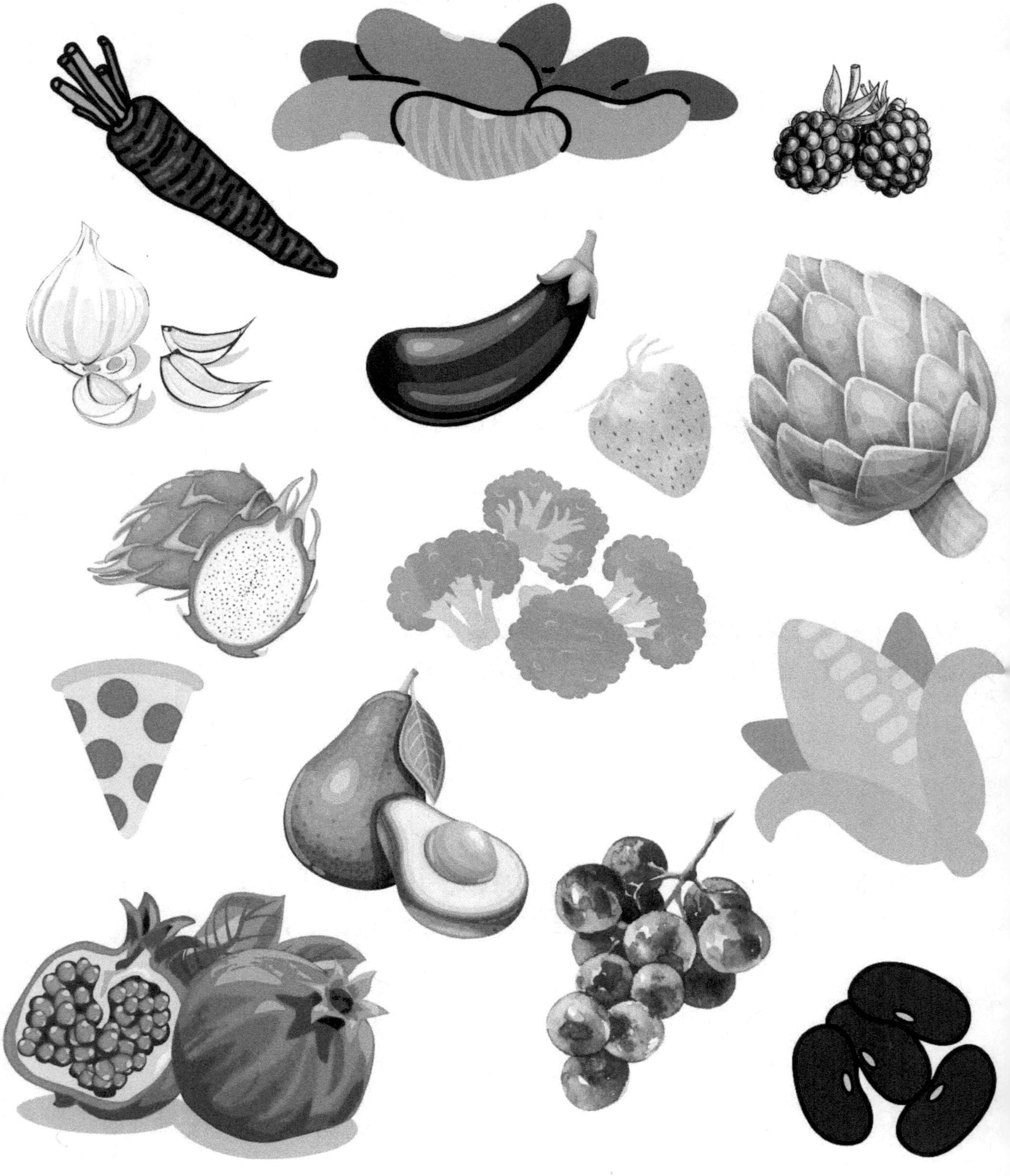

Superfoods

List at least 10 more superfoods and describe their super power properties.

Practice your cursive handwriting skills!

Write a comic about a battle between healthy vs. unhealthy foods.

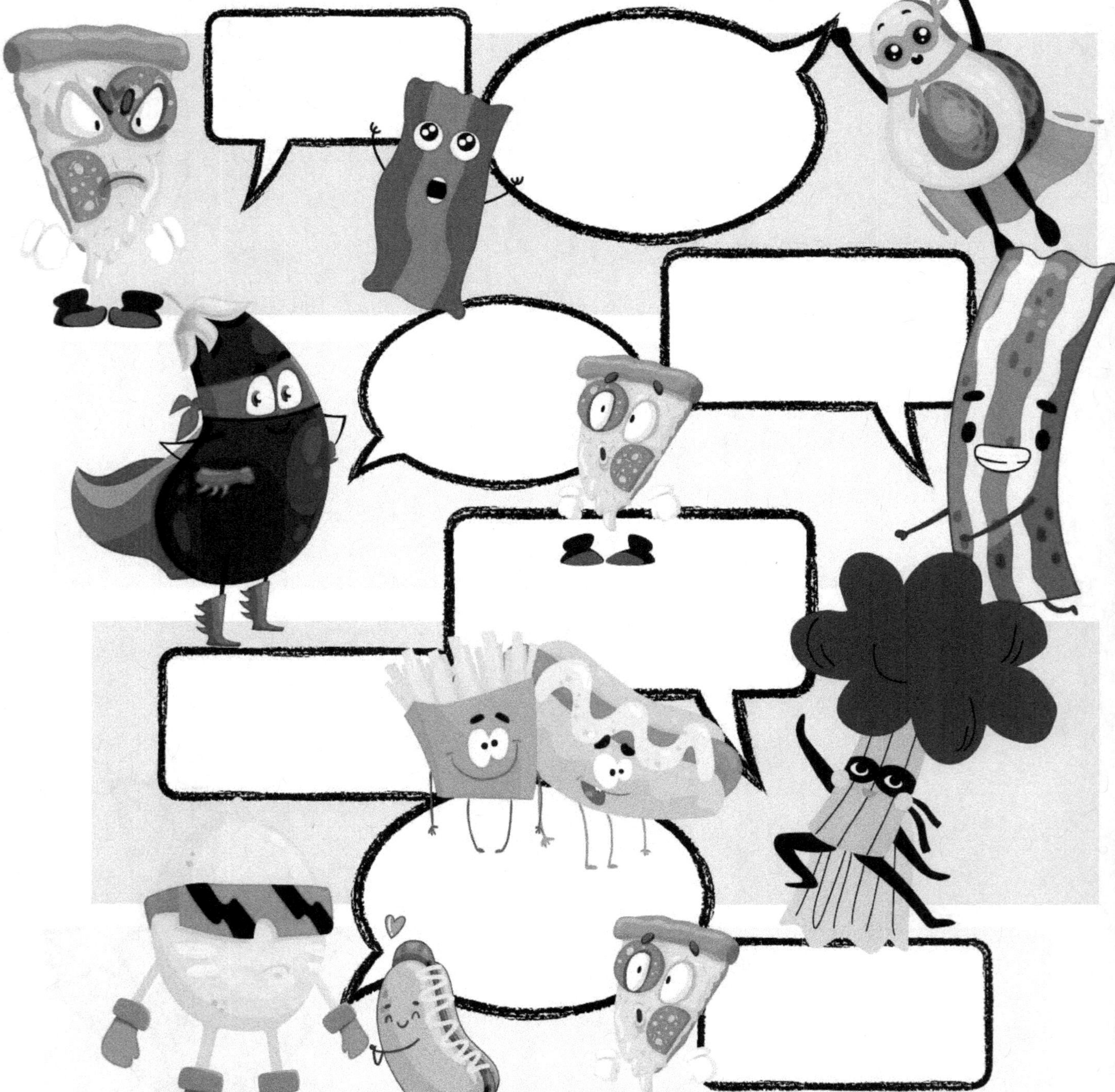

Your turn to make another comic! Draw your superfood heroes.

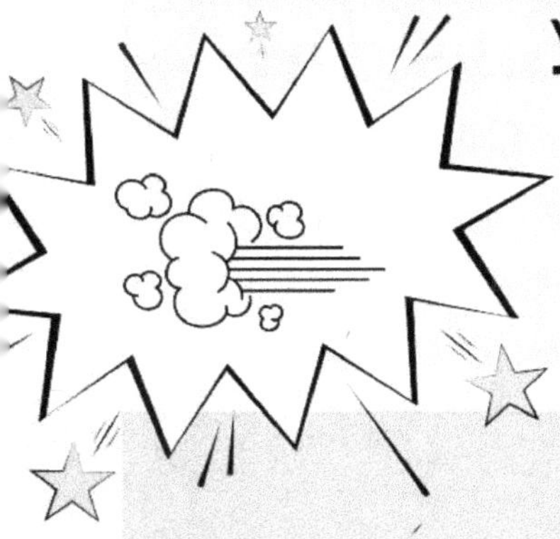

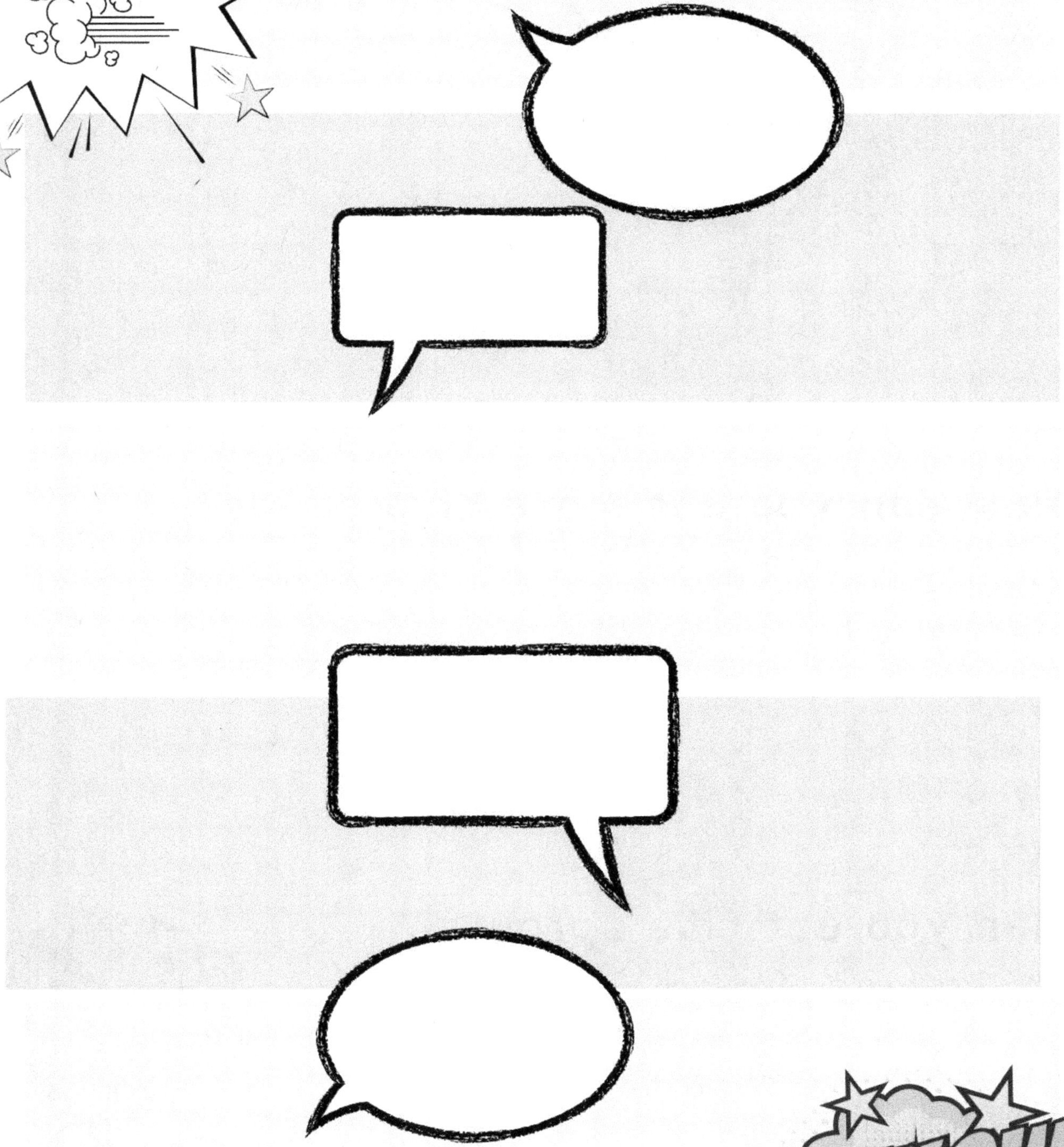

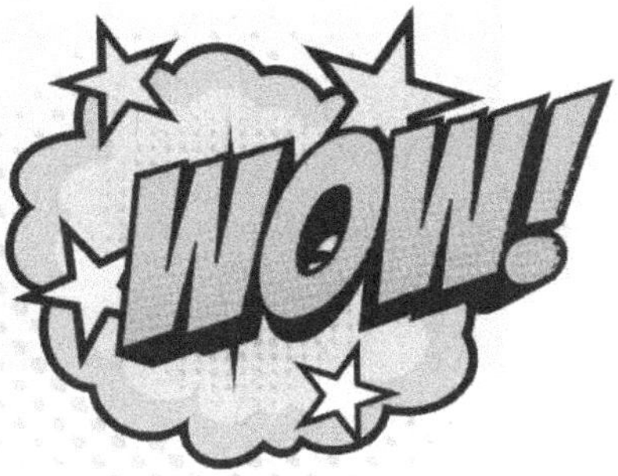

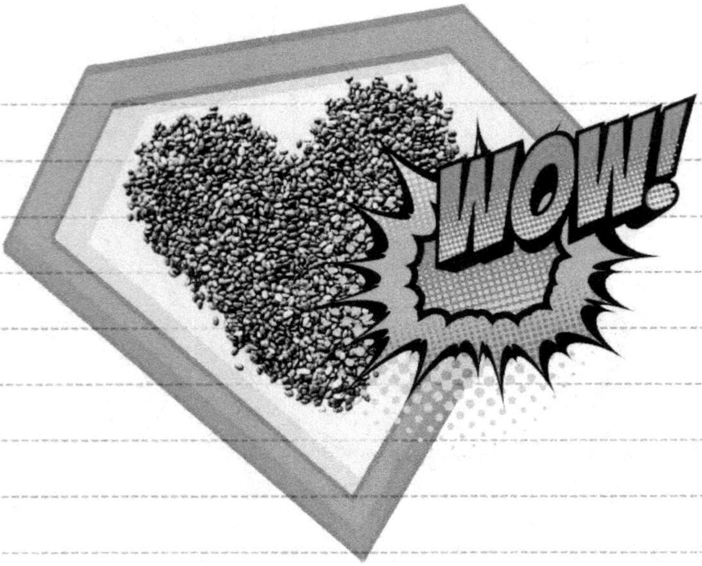

Discuss the super power of chia seeds.

How can you eat more chia seeds?

Can you eat chia sprouts?

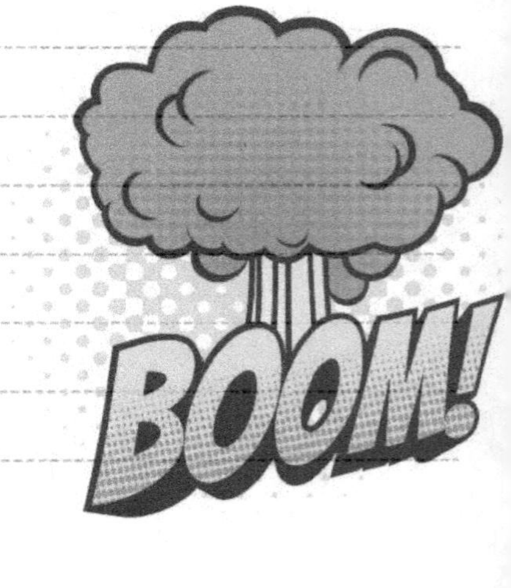

The Chia Scrambler

Unscramble this superfood recipe and rewrite the final copy on the following page. Research the steps to this simple chia pudding recipe if needed.

Ingredients

Stir chia seeds and honey into puree. Refrigerate for 4 hours. Puree strawberries and milk together. Grab a spoon, eat, and enjoy! Pour strawberry milk puree in small bowls or cups.

Directions

1 cup fresh strawberries, hulled
1 cup nut milk or regular milk
1/4 cup chia seeds
1 Tablespoon honey (optional)

Chia Pudding Recipe

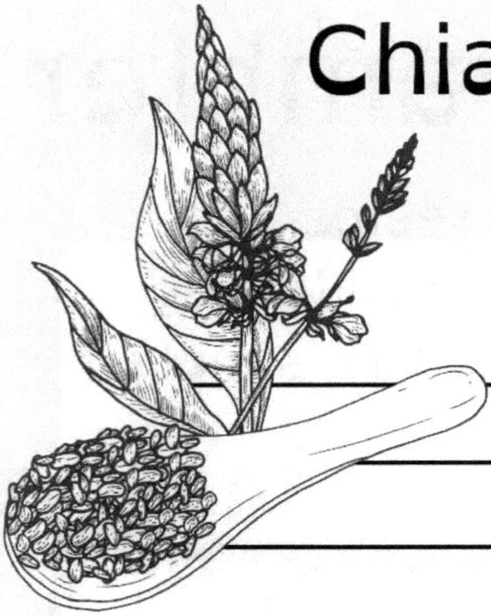

Ingredients

Yield: Cost: Time:

Directions

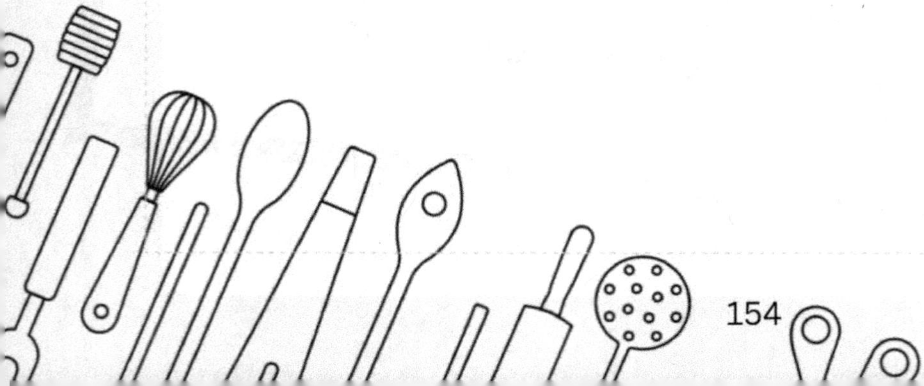

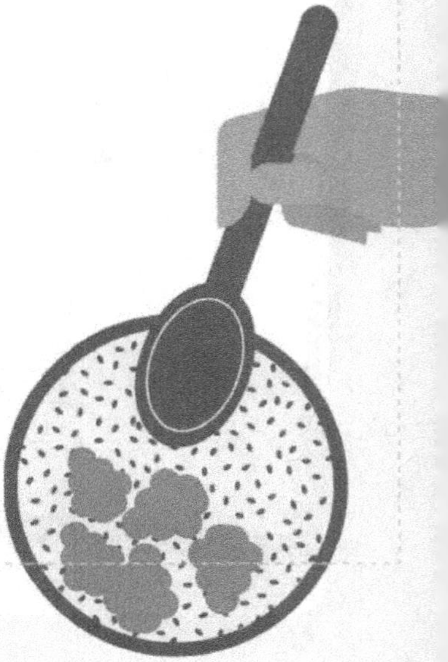

Br-Avocado!

Find the top fifteen most popular avocados in the word search below.

B	V	I	P	L	A	E	A	R	J	Y	N	U	H	Q
G	R	O	B	N	O	R	M	B	G	Y	E	O	N	B
K	N	Q	L	R	F	X	U	T	G	E	I	Z	R	F
F	R	Y	N	U	I	T	L	Y	N	R	T	O	I	S
A	U	O	H	R	L	R	A	E	E	E	G	I	C	D
L	M	E	D	C	E	A	M	E	F	D	W	O	L	L
I	A	O	R	X	R	G	D	G	E	P	O	G	E	I
V	O	N	A	T	U	Z	N	N	P	T	H	H	O	W
H	Z	C	Q	U	E	V	P	I	Y	G	X	A	P	R
U	N	C	H	O	Q	U	E	T	T	E	B	S	A	A
V	S	Z	S	P	A	T	G	R	B	T	E	S	T	H
Z	P	G	W	U	J	V	O	W	X	A	E	N	R	S
G	K	K	R	S	Y	X	K	J	F	O	S	Q	A	P
W	R	Y	W	S	W	F	H	T	T	B	A	C	O	N
N	O	T	R	E	K	N	I	P	B	Z	F	H	J	I

Lula **Pinkerton** **Bacon**
Gwen **Choquette** **Maluma**
Hass **Cleopatra** **Monroe**
Fuerte **Ettinger** **Brogden**
Reed **Zutano** **Sharwil**

What are some of the top reasons avocados are so super?

Do avocados have more potassium than bananas?

What is potassium and how is it good for the body?

Are avocados rich in fats?

Explain the difference between healthy fats and unhealthy fats.

Name a few other types of healthy fats and what foods have them.

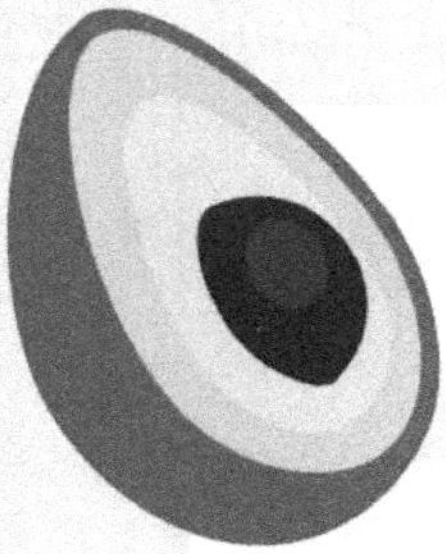

Supercado Spa

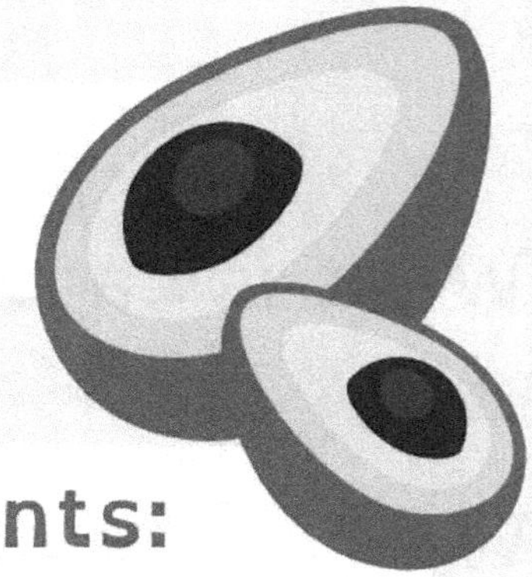

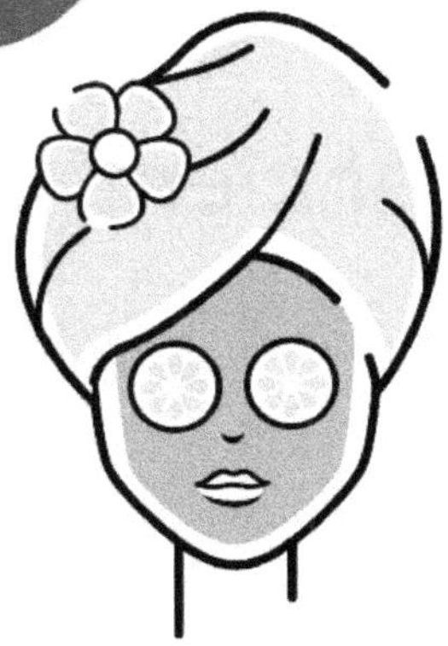

Ingredients:

1/2 cup Ripe Avocado
3 Tablespoons of Honey
2 Cucumber Slices

Directions:

- In a small bowl, mash avocado until smooth.
- Add the honey and stir well.
- Apply mixture on your face, avoiding the eye areas.
- Lay on your back and place the cucumber slices over your eyes.
- Breathe and relax for the next 10 minutes. **SPA TIP:** Play relaxing music, practice meditation, breathing techniques, or even say a positive affirmation while waiting for the mask to work into the skin.
- After ten minutes, rinse.
- Enjoy freshly hydrated skin!

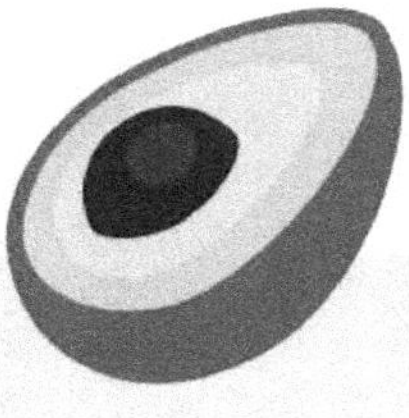

Superfood Cacao

What is cacao?

Was cacao used as a currency in ancient days? Explain.

Is cacao rich in iron, magnesium, or calcium?

Compare these amounts to other foods.

What recipes would you want to make with cacao?

What is carob powder and how does it relate to cacao? Is it a superfood too?

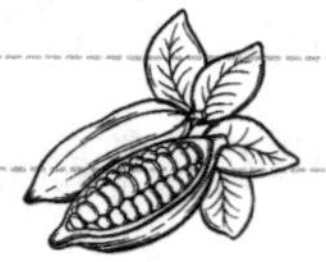

Cacao vs. Cocoa vs. Carob

Explain the differences between the three.

Cacao	Cocoa	Carob

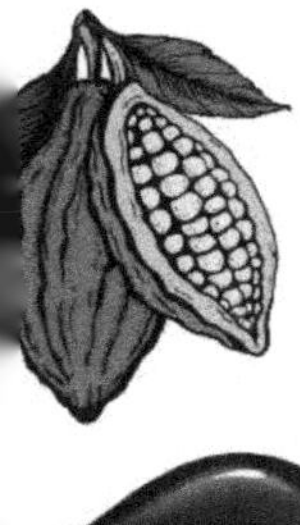

CACAO *Smoothie*

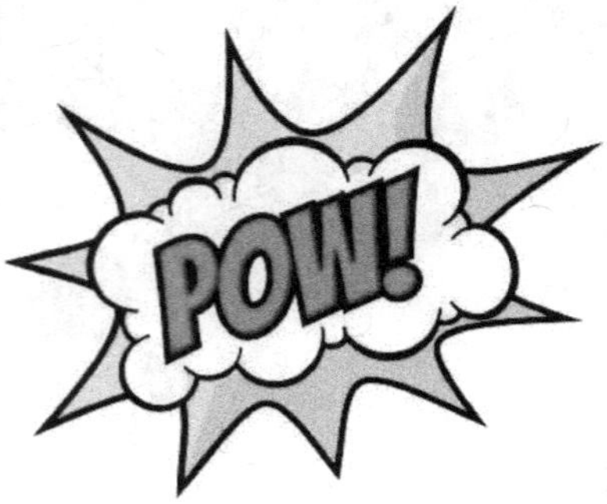

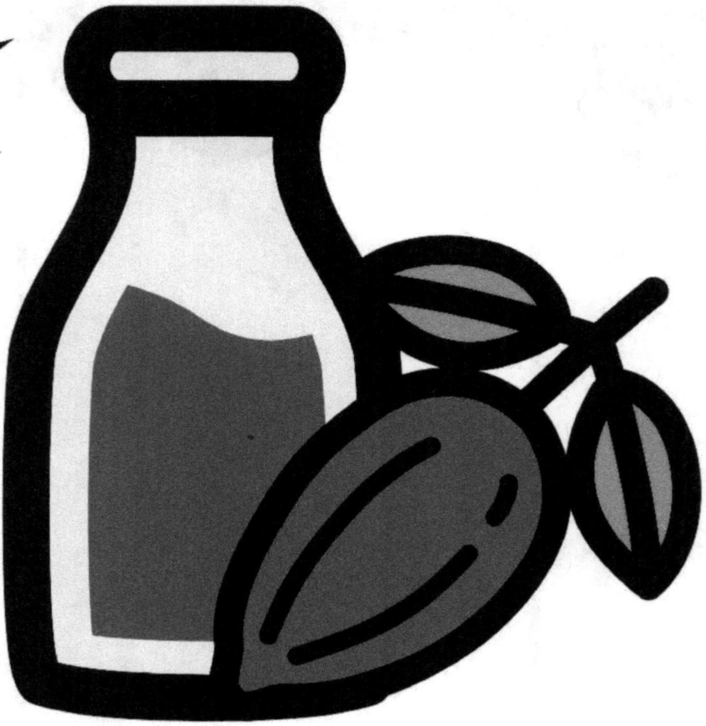

INGREDIENTS

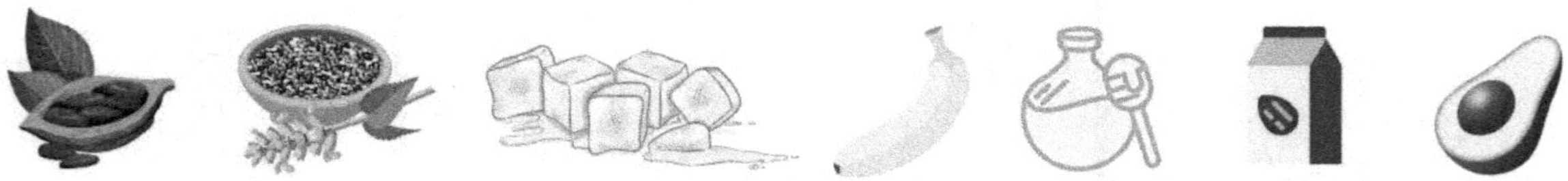

Cacao | Chia Seeds | Ice Cubes | Banana | Honey | Nut Milk | Avocado

BLEND TOGETHER & ENJOY

2 Tablespoons Cacao 1 Tablespoon Chia Seeds 1/2 cup Ice Cubes 1 Banana, peeled & frozen	1 Tablespoon Honey 2 cups Nut Milk or other Milk 1/2 Avocado, peeled & no seed

Smoothie Reflection Time

Did you enjoy this recipe?

Did you notice an increase of energy from the cacao?

Could you taste the avocado?
Was the consistency just right?

Could you feel the chia seeds, or did the blender liquify them?

Would you make any changes to the ingredients?

By naming a few health benefits this drink has, how could you describe, advertise, influence, or suggest this healthy drink to others?

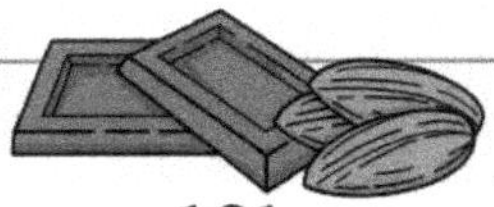

Rewrite your version of the recipe, making changes to quantities, steps, ingredients, or anything else you find fitting.

Recipe Name

Procedure

Yield

Cost

Time

Ingredients

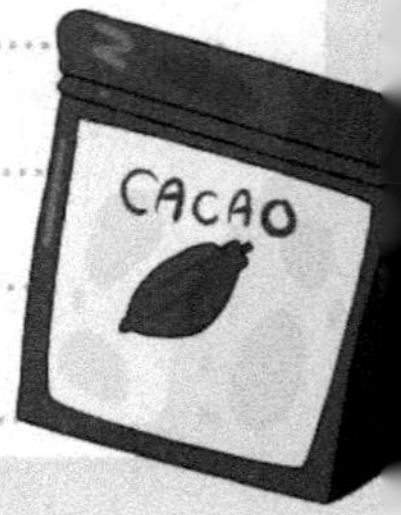

How much would you charge for 16 oz?

What is your profit margin?

A MINERAL MINE

Antioxidant Alley

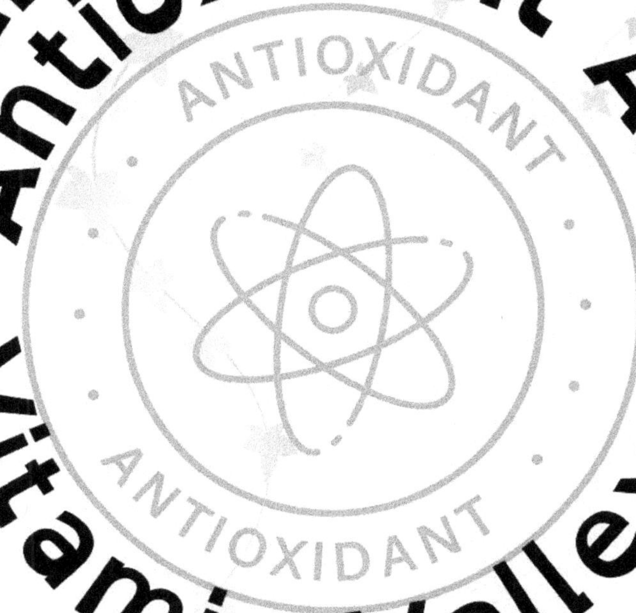

Vitamin Valley

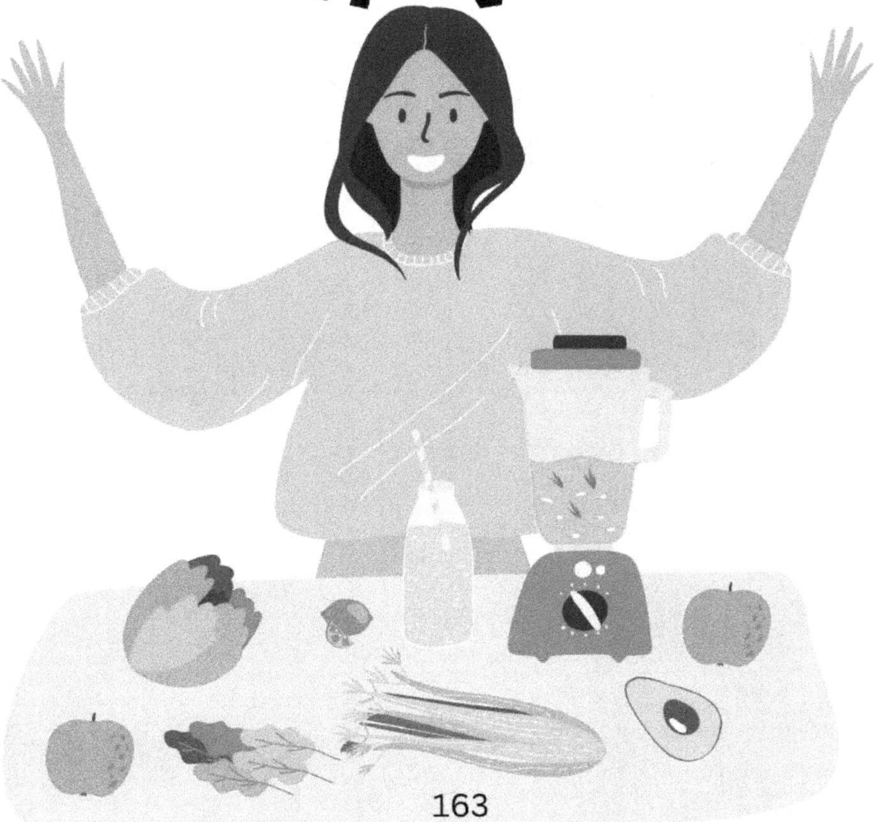

Explain what an antioxidant is and what it does.

What are the similarities and differences between vitamins, minerals, and antioxidants?

What are some vitamin, mineral, and antioxidant rich foods and beverages? How could you include these in your daily meal plan?

Discuss synthetic vitamins, minerals, antioxidants. Can they provide the same benefits as the antioxidants derived from food sources?

What is phytic acid?

What foods are rich in phytic acids?

How does phytic acid disrupt absorption of vitamins and minerals?

Discuss the benefits of these **vitamins** and which foods they are abundant in.

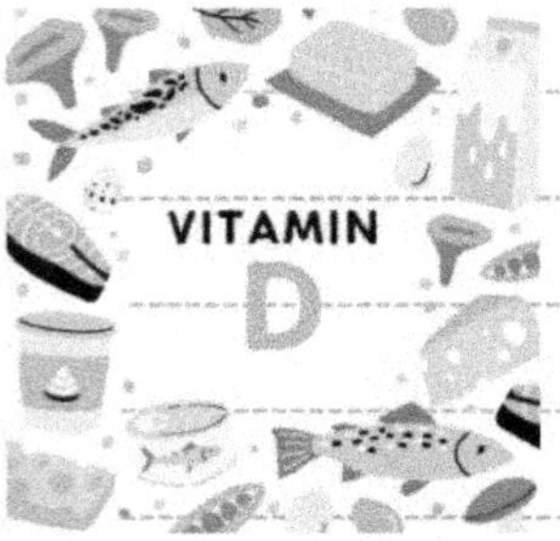

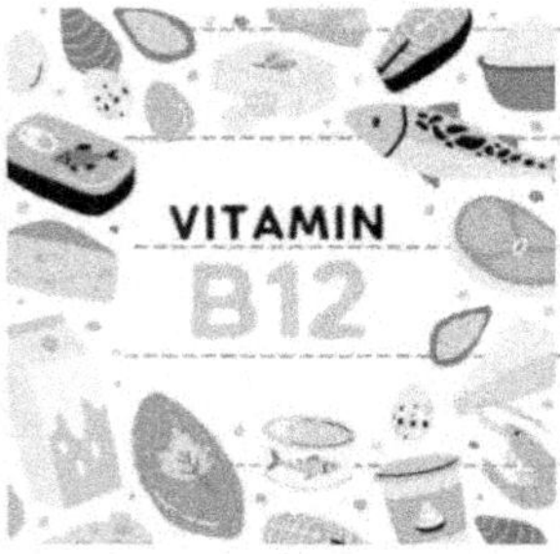

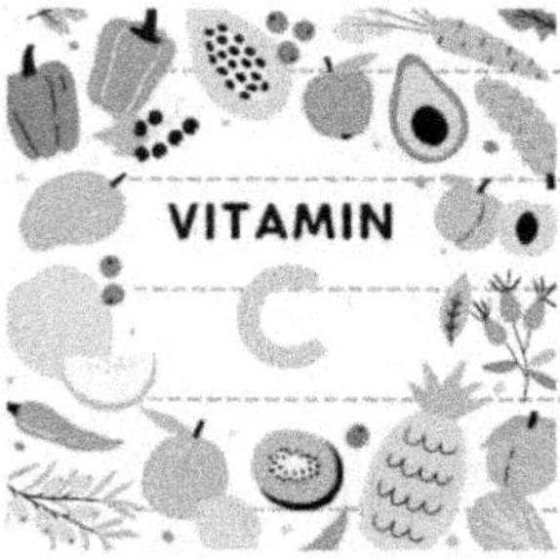

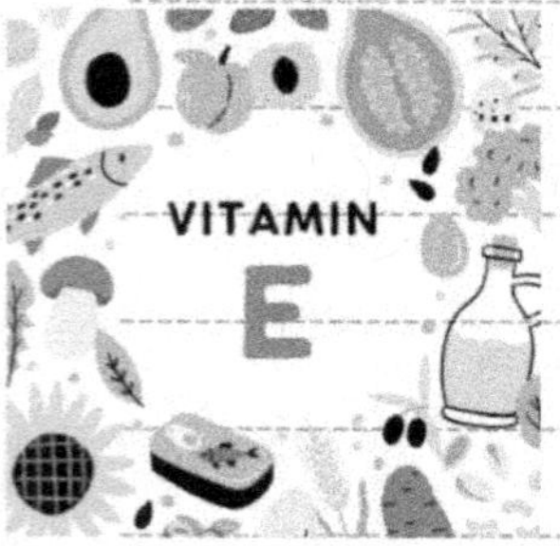

Practice your cursive handwriting skills!

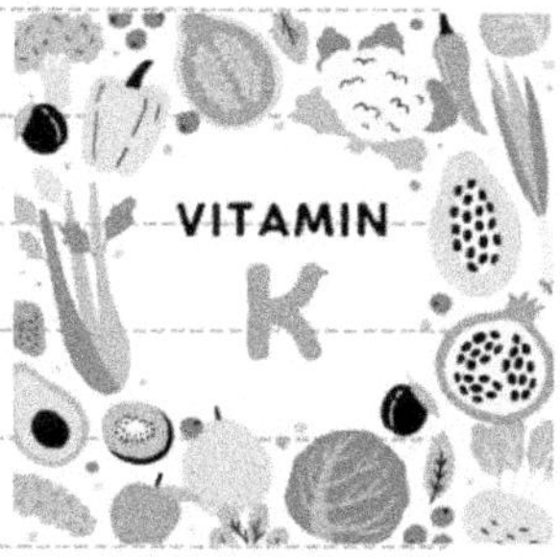

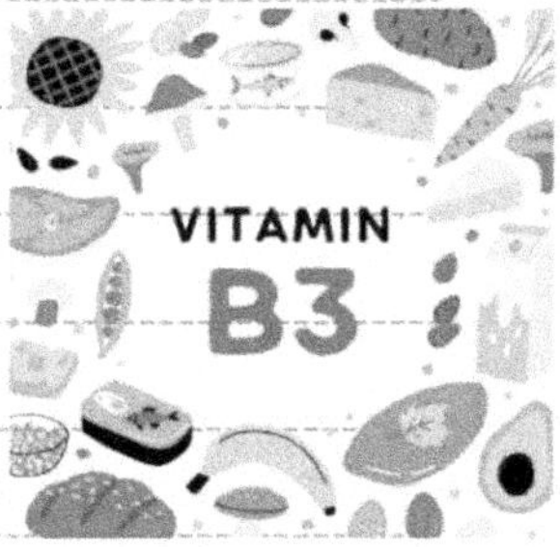

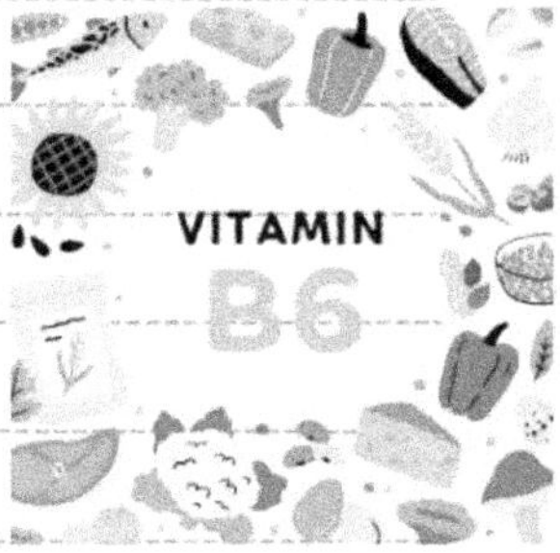

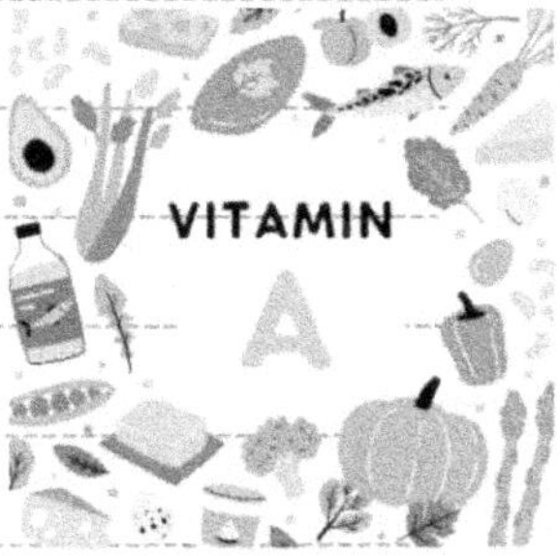

Draw some of your favorite vitamin, mineral, and antioxidant rich foods.

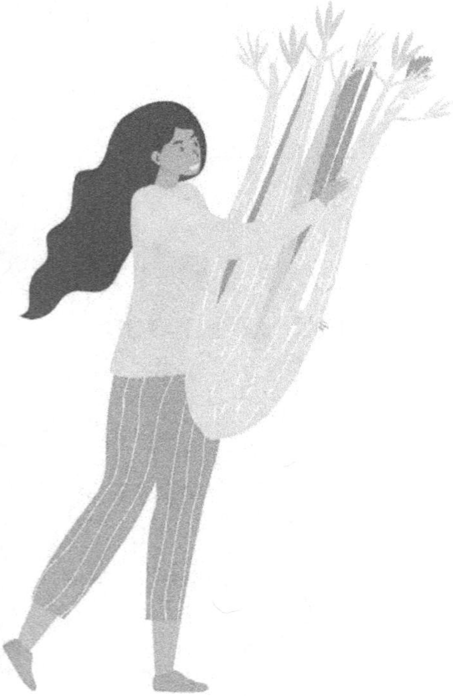

ALLEY, VALLEY, & MINE

Research and write down the antioxidant, vitamin, and mineral properties.

PINEAPPLE

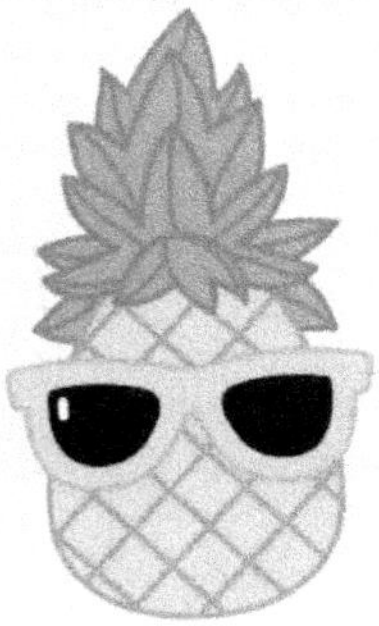

Rich in potassium, calcium, vitamin C, K, B6, magnesium, phosphorus, as well as soluble and insoluble fiber.

WATERMELON

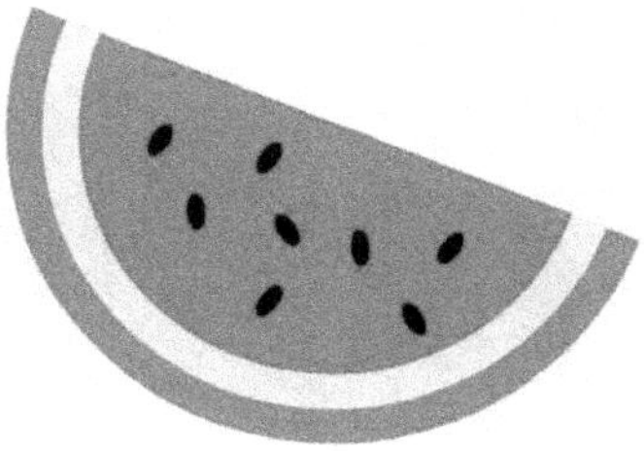

KALE

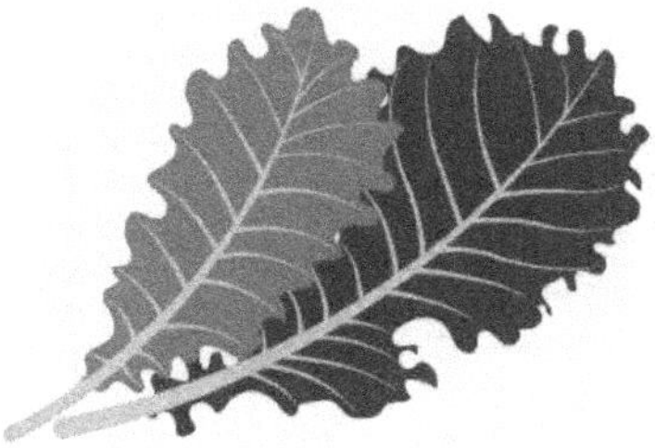

LEMON

POMEGRANATE

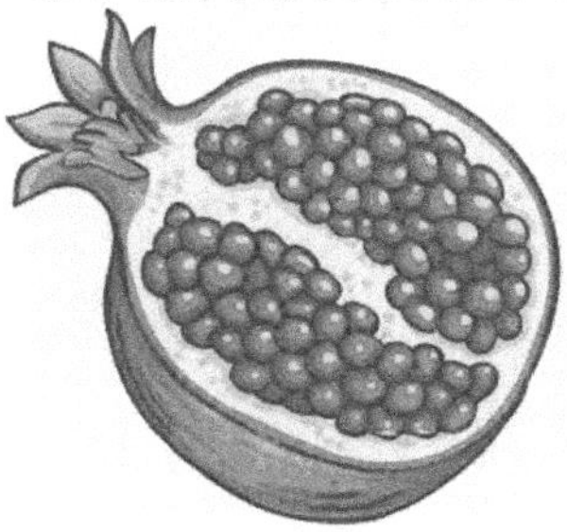

GARLIC

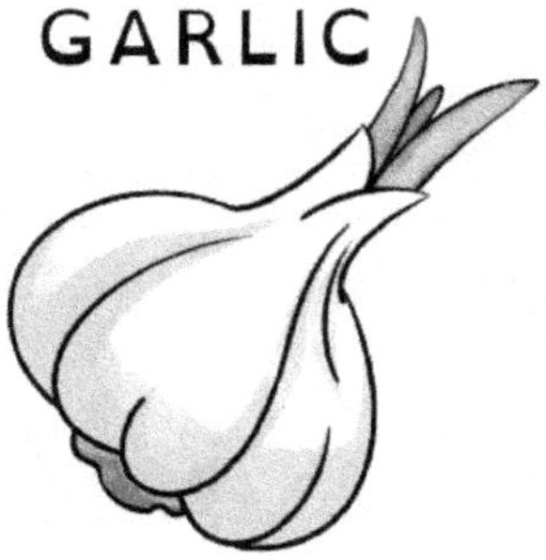

ALLEY, VALLEY, & MINE

Research and write down the antioxidant, vitamin, and mineral properties.

CHERRY

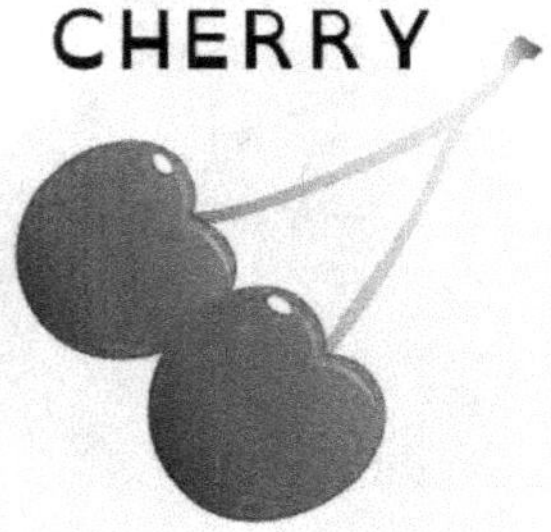

EGGPLANT

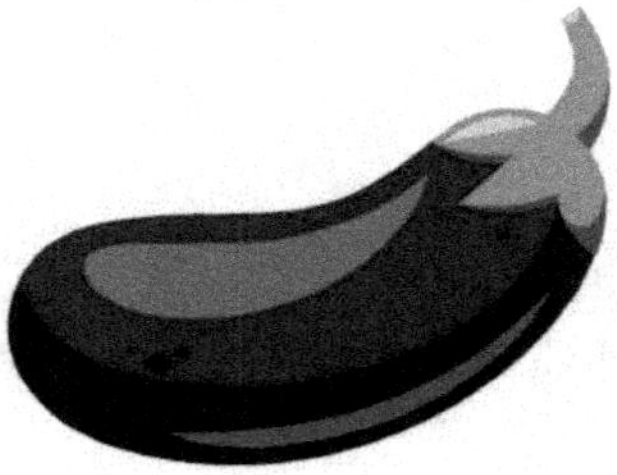

AVOCADO

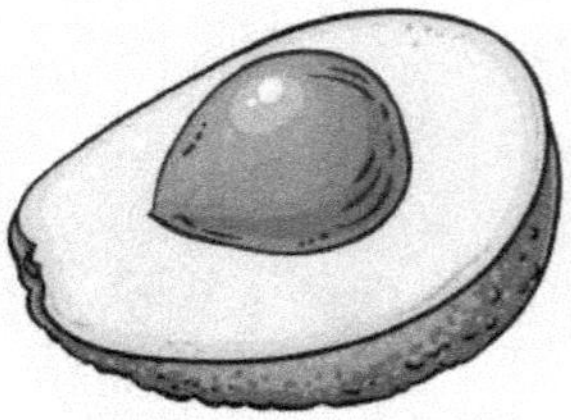

CARROT

KIWI

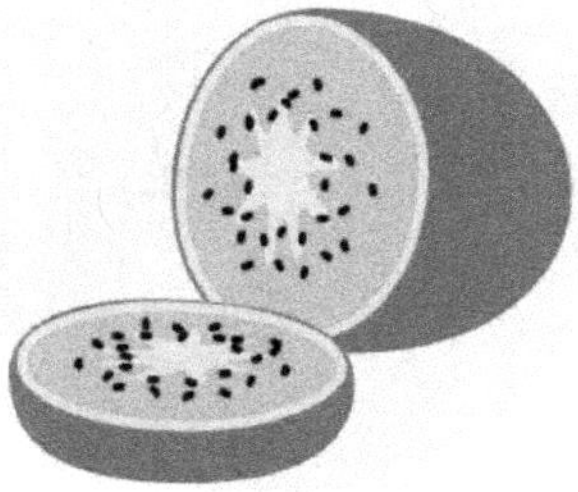

BEET

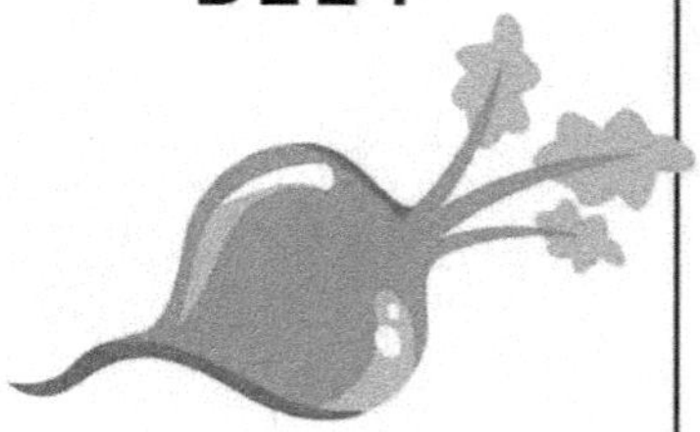

ALLEY, VALLEY, & MINE

Research and write down the antioxidant, vitamin, and mineral properties.

LEMON

Has nourishing elements like vitamin C, vitamin B6, vitamin A, vitamin E, folate, niacin thiamin, and riboflavin.

PUMPKIN

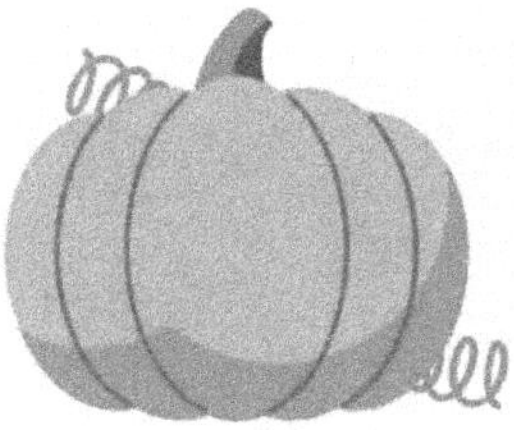

ARTICHOKE

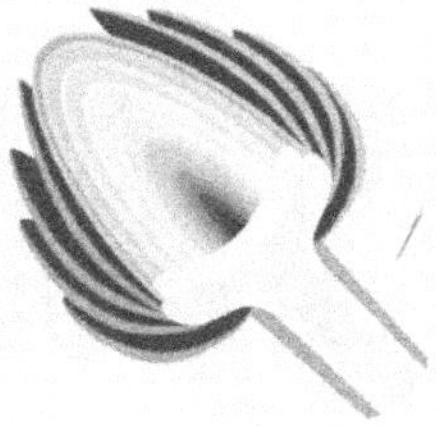

BROCCOLI

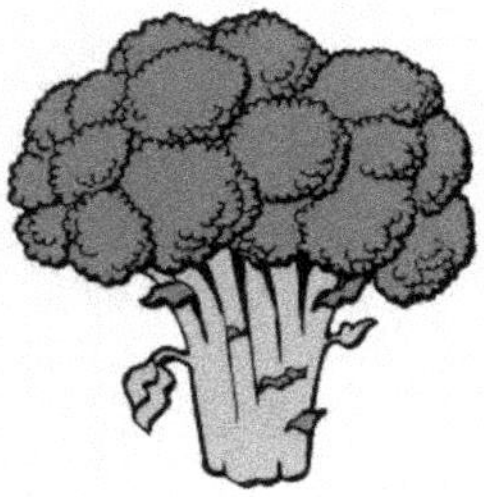

BLUEBERRIES

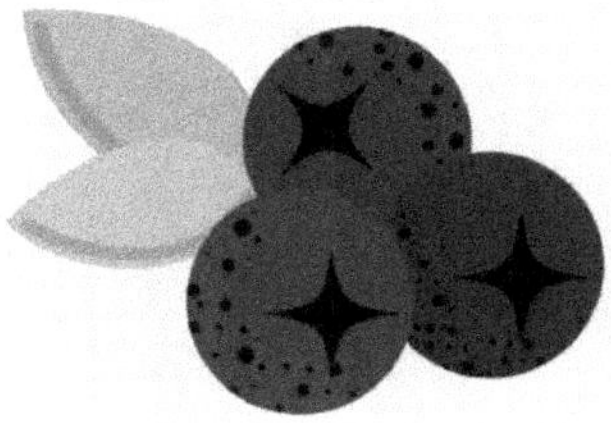

CABBAGE

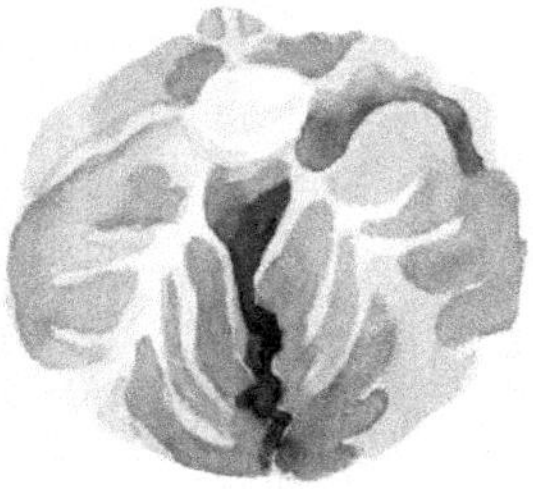

ALLEY, VALLEY, & MINE

Research and write down the antioxidant, vitamin, and mineral properties.

GRAPES

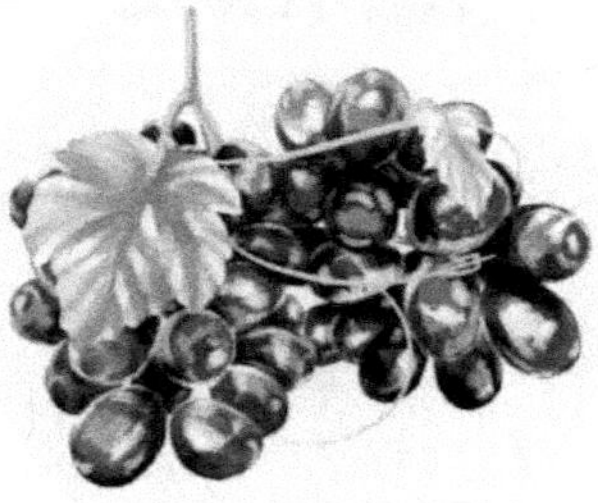

SPINACH

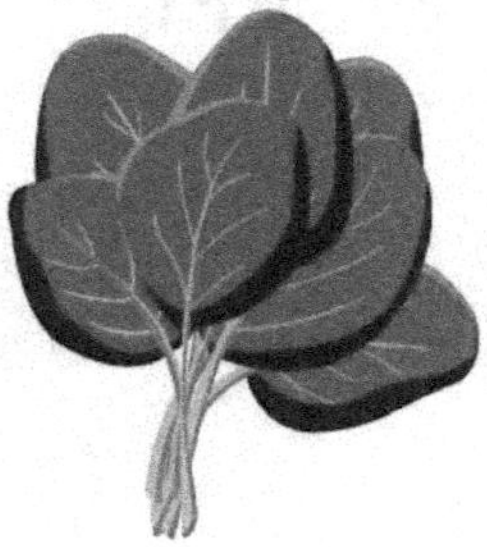

STRAWBERRY

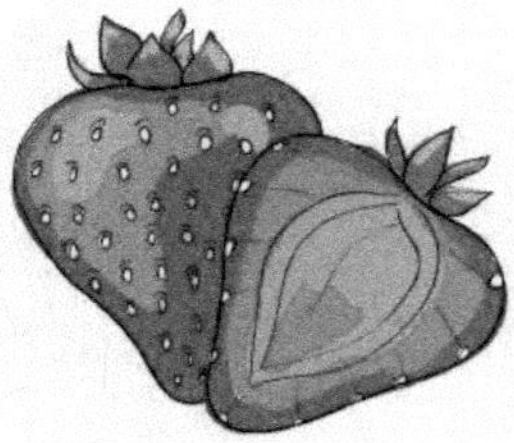

PARSNIPS

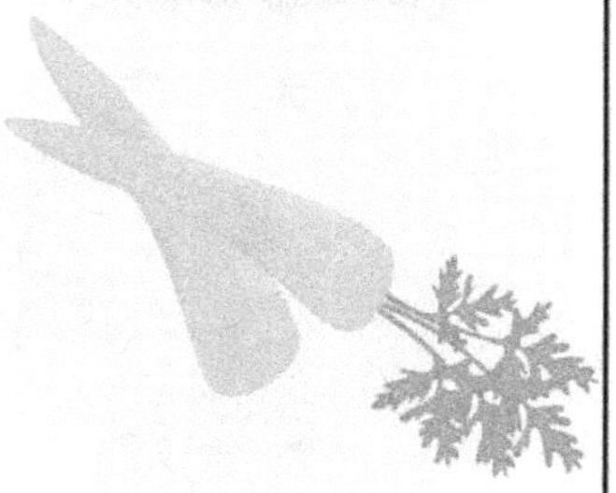

GUAVA

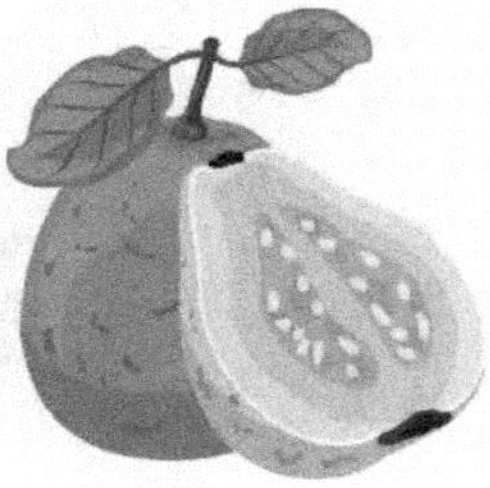

FENNEL

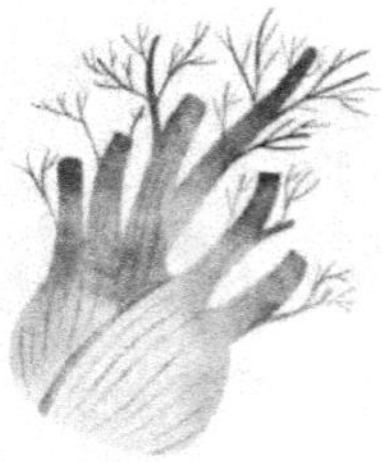

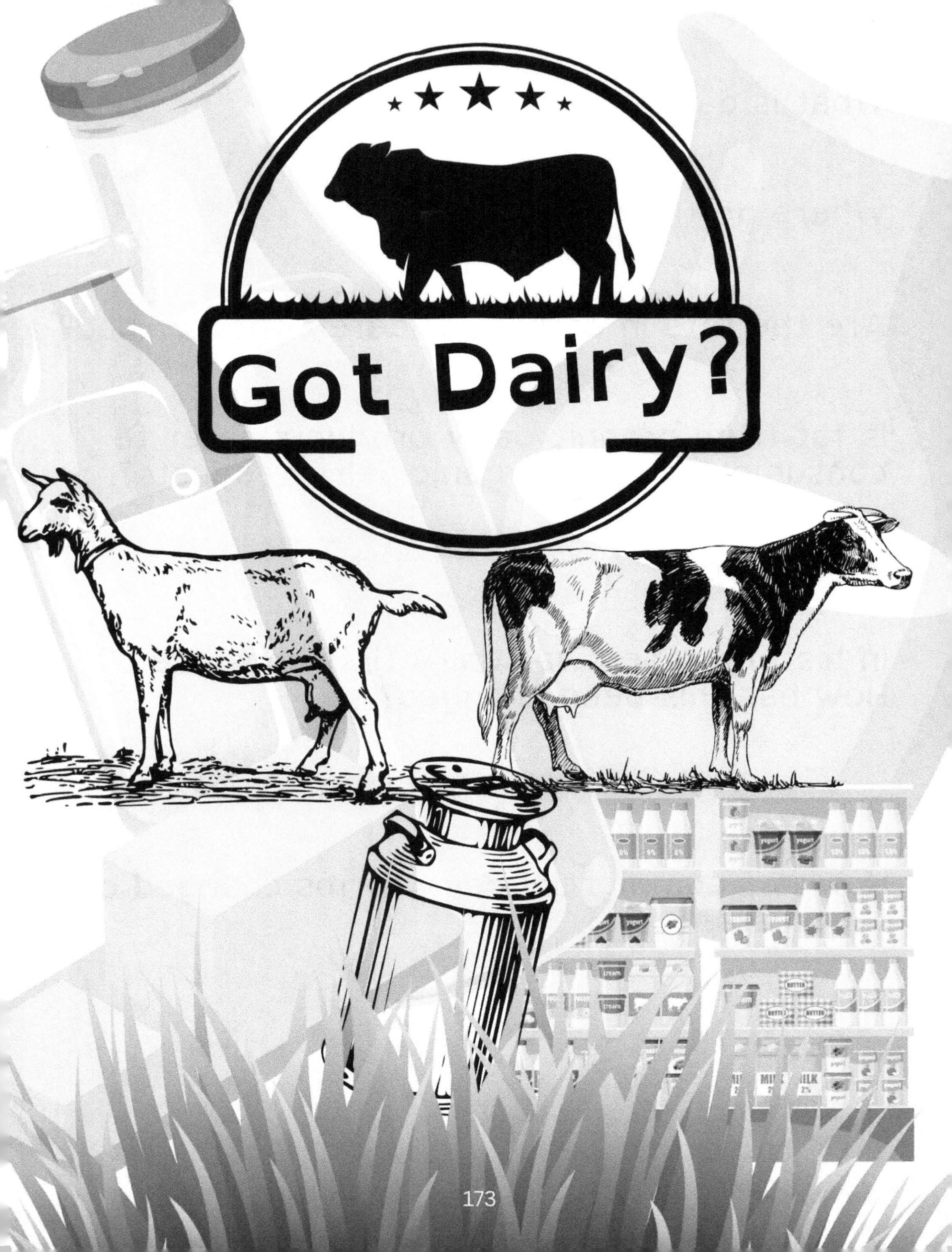
Got Dairy?

What is dairy? What is lactose?

Where do they come from?

Are the fats in dairy considered good or bad?

Is fat from organic dairy products safer to consume than non-organic dairy products?

In history, when was dairy first consumed? How has this been changed?

How has commercial dairy farms changed over the years?

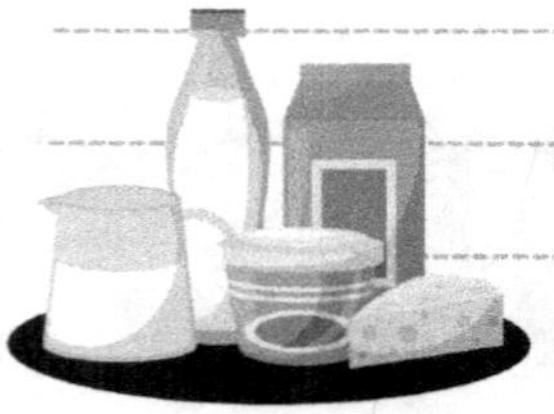

When babies are born, what do they consume? Why? Is milk important in our diet?

What kind of animals produce milk?

What nutrients are in milk?

What are some some things to consider when buying milk and dairy? Example: Research added hormones, antibiotics, raw milk, organic, grass fed, humane practices, etc.

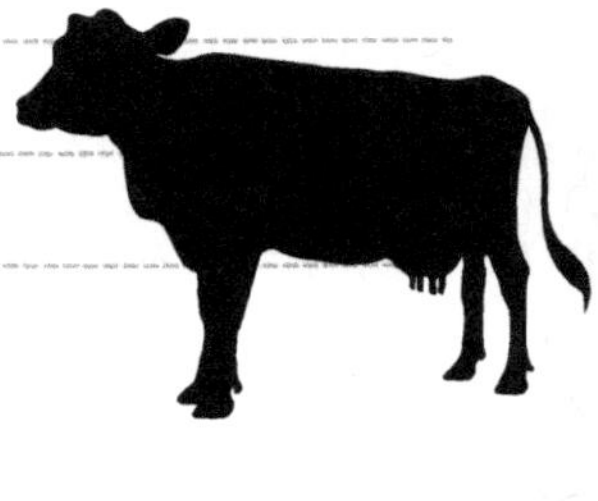

Where do you get your dairy products?

Take a minute and research the company or companies you get your dairy from. Write what you learn: Who? What? When? Why? Where? How?

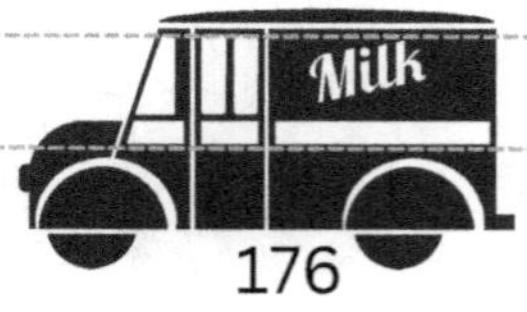

Take some time to research, draw, and label what makes a happy grass fed dairy farm.

Do you think when you consume dairy from a happy cow that this can make a difference in your body, mood, and absorption? Research and explain. Bonus: compare your mood when consuming each type of milk/dairy products.

What is Dairy Free dairy?

Who and why would someone choose dairy free products?

Can vegetarians have dairy?

How about vegans?

List a few alternatives to dairy.

The Nut Milk Scrambler

Unscramble the recipe and rewrite the final copy on the following page. Research the steps to this simple nut recipe if needed.

Ingredients

Drain. Pour nut blend through cheese cloth or nut milk bag. Refrigerate. Soak nuts for 3 hours in 3 cups of filtered water. Blend soaked nuts with 4 cups of cold filtered water. Enjoy your fresh and cold nut milk!

Directions

1 cup raw, unsalted nuts
3 cups filtered water
4 cups cold filtered water

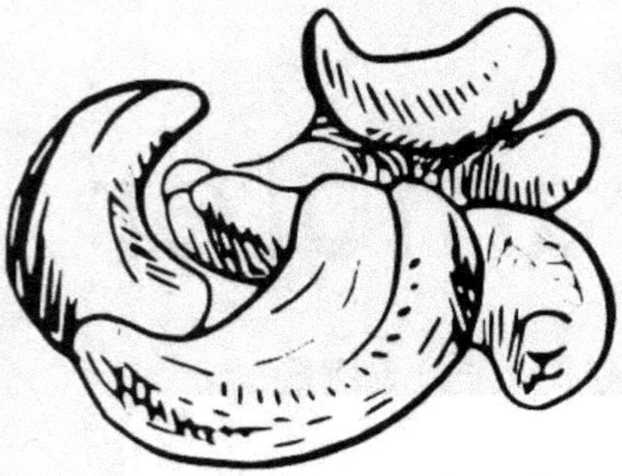

Delicious Nut Milk Recipe

Ingredients

Yield: Cost: Time:

Directions

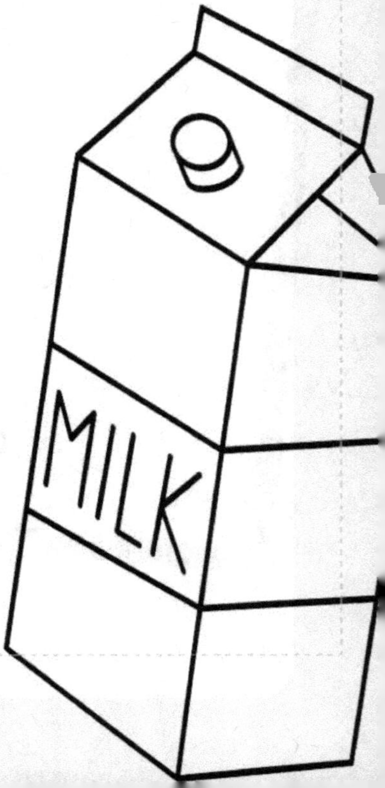

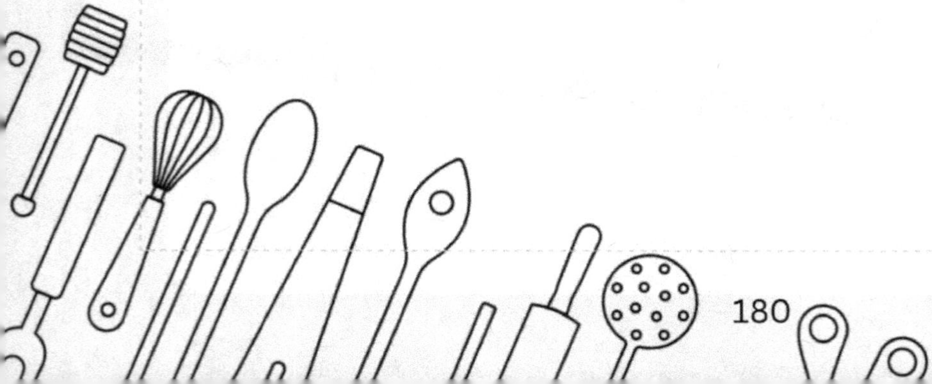

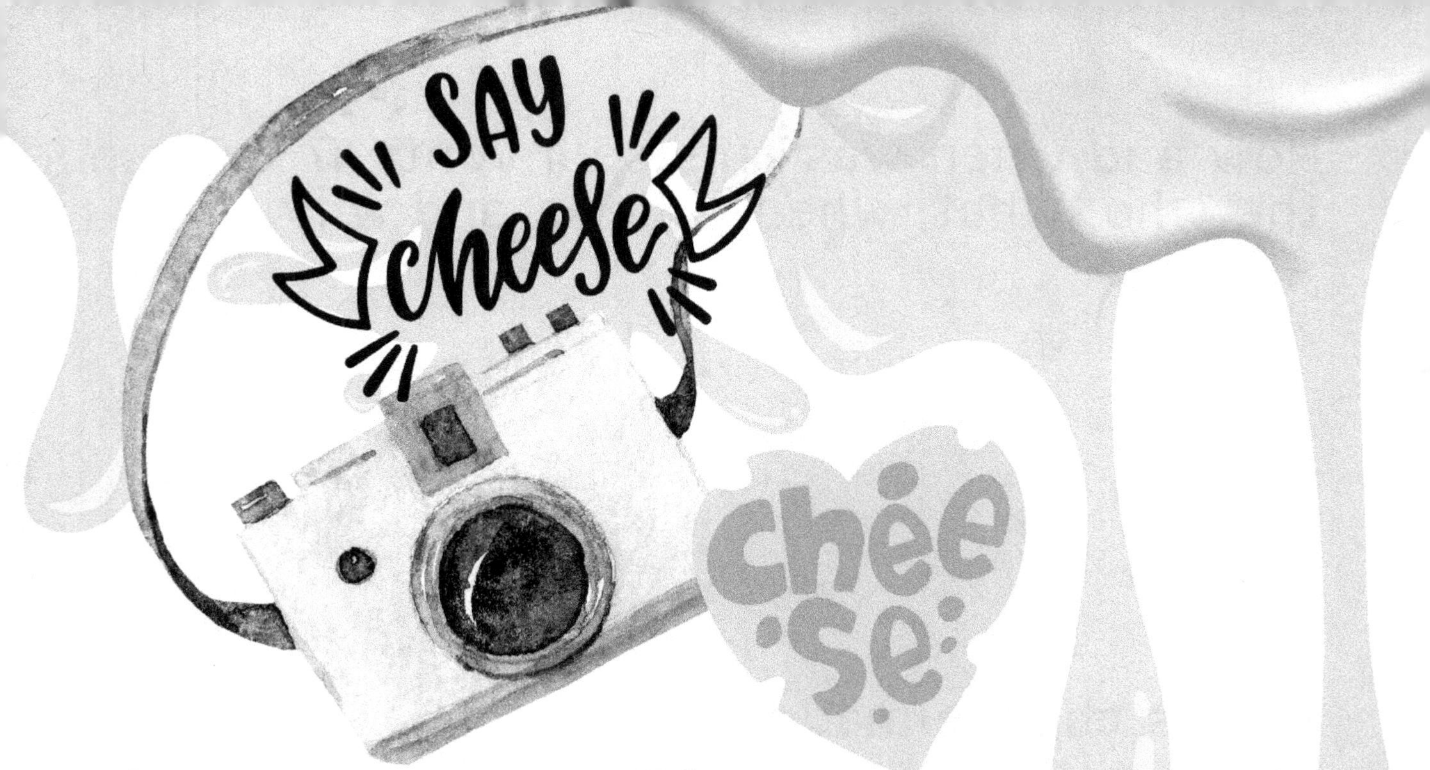

Get Some Cheesy Jokes!

Who cut the cheese?
Find and make your own cheesy jokes.

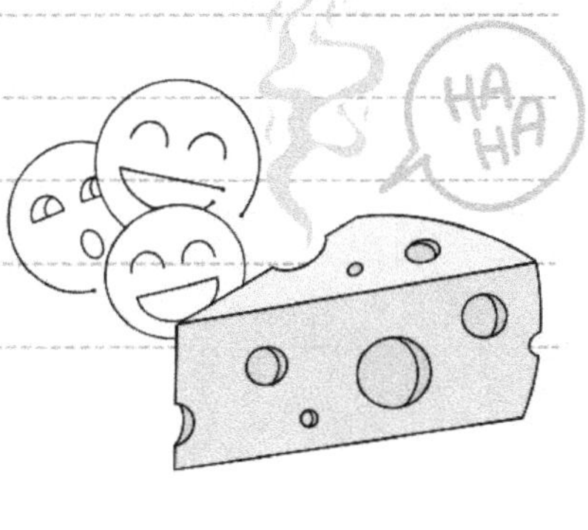

How and when was cheese invented? Explain the who, what, when, where, and why.

How is cheese made?

How are the vegan or dairy free alternatives different?

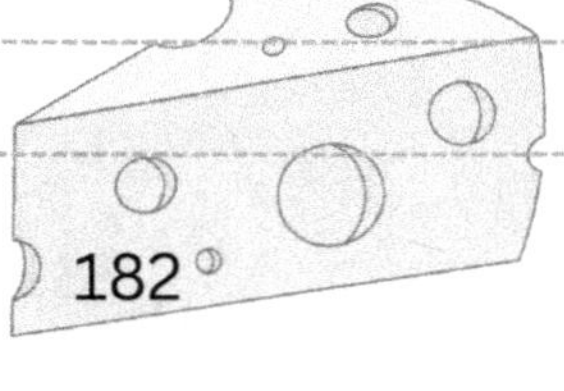

Why is cheese stinky?

Why are there holes in Swiss cheese?

Why are some cheeses yellow and others white or blue?

Why are some cheeses soft and others hard?

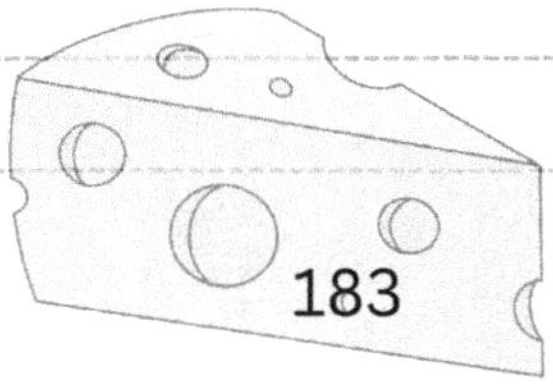

Name as many cheeses as you can find. Which ones have you tried? How long does each cheese take to make? Label your favorites and least favorites.

Practice your cursive handwriting skills!

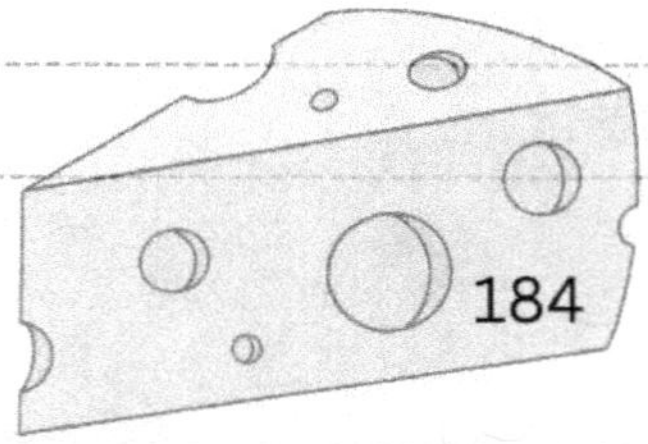

Butter on the Move!
How does butter move?

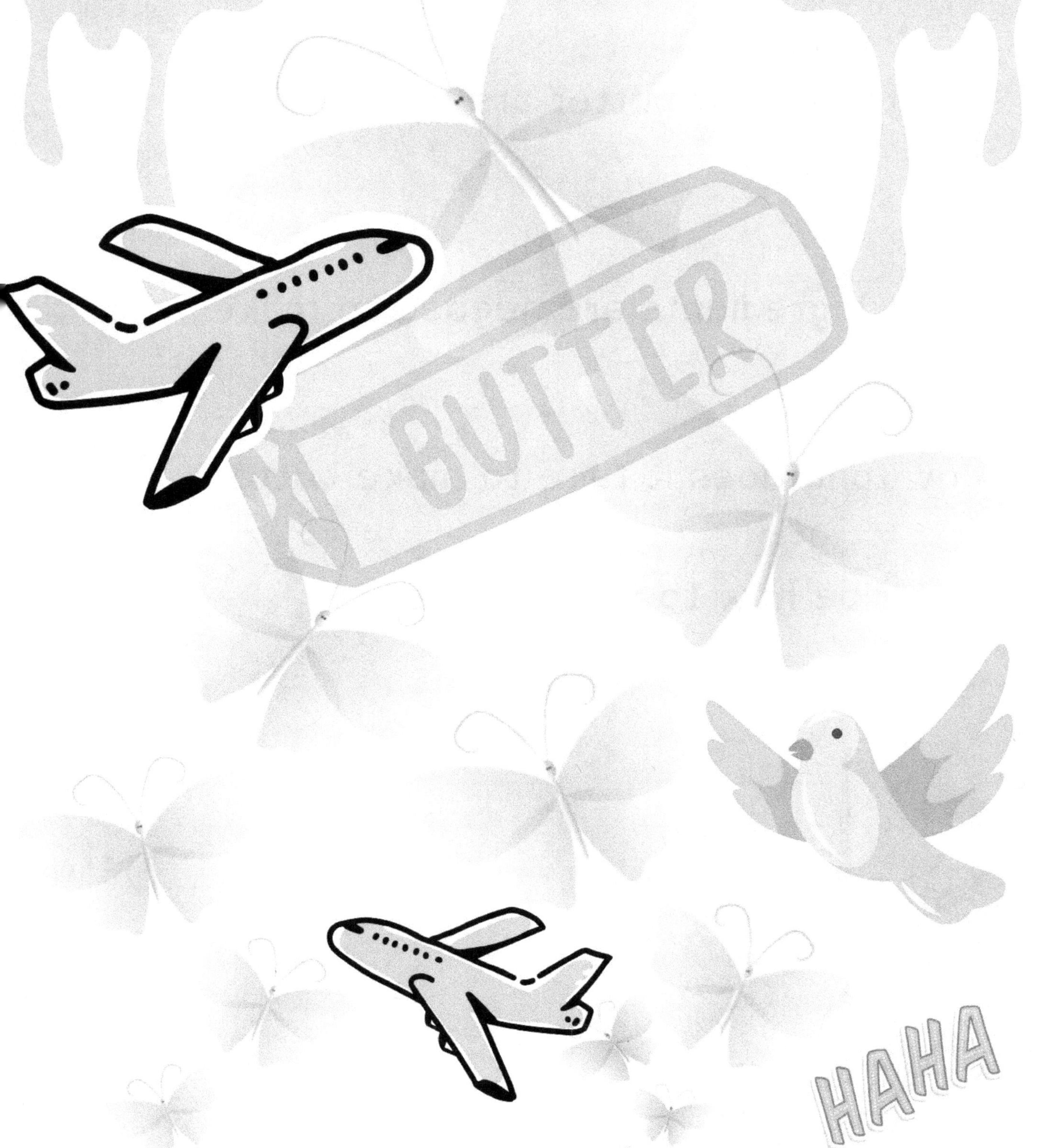

What is butter made from?

What types of butter are there?

What ingredients are needed to make butter?

How long does it take to make butter?

Describe how to make butter.

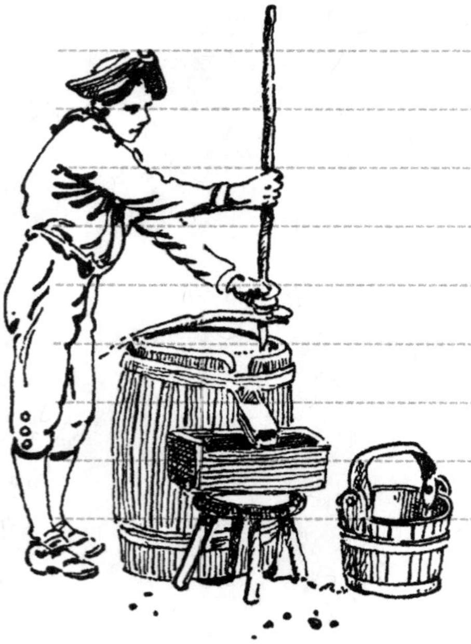

Why are cultures added to butter?

What is left behind when the cream turns to butter?

Why was adding salt to butter important before refrigeration was common?

Have you had homemade butter before? Describe the differences. If not make some!

What is a dairy free/vegan option of traditional butter?

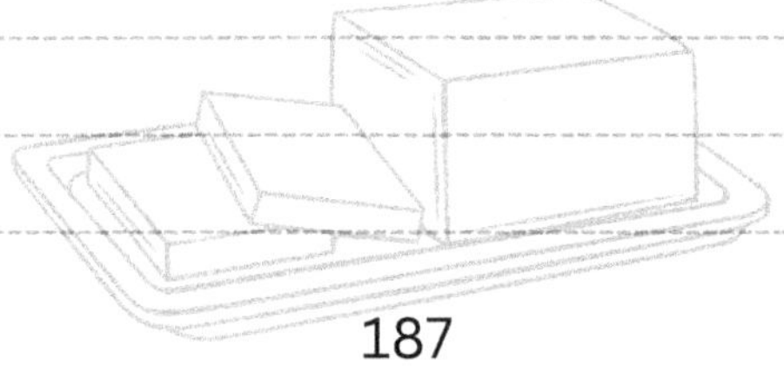

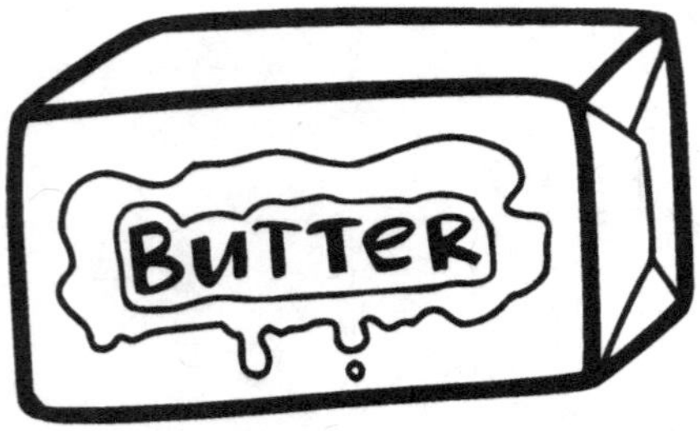

Butter Math

The fat percentage in heavy cream makes a difference when making butter. The higher the fat content, the more butter and less buttermilk your end result will be. Rule of thumb, no less than 35% fat in your heavy cream to make butter. How do you know the percentage of fat? Most of the time it is not labeled directly on the package. This is where a little mathematician brain comes in. Find the percentage of fat content for this heavy cream (needed information is located on the 'Nutrition Facts' label on carton:

Calories per serving (35)
Total fat per serving (2g)
Hint: (1g of fat = 9 calories)

Is this worth making butter from?

How is yogurt made?

Give a step by step procedure of how yogurt is made, from start to finish.

Practice your cursive handwriting skills!

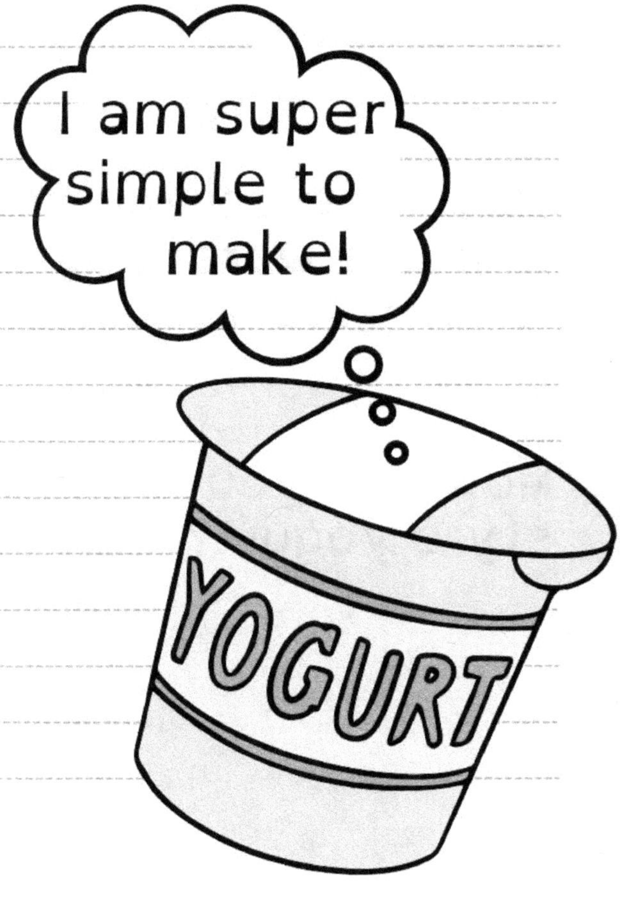

Explain the difference in procedures when making Greek yogurt.

Do you need to pasteurize your milk before you use it to make yogurt?

At what temperature is pasteurization achieved?

What is in raw milk, that is not in pasteurized milk?

What temperature do you add your culture in at? Explain.

How long do you need to keep your milk mixture warm and at what temperature untill it turns to yogurt?

How can you make thicker yogurt, like greek style yogurt?

Probiotics

What are probiotics and what do they do?

Where can you find them?

Are probiotics in all dairy and fermented foods?

What are "live cultures"?

List several benefits of probiotics.

Name a few dairy free yogurt alternatives. Do they have probiotics in them? Explain.

Power of Gut Health

Look up these words. Write down what they are and how they can effect your health and mood.

Insoluble Fiber

Prebiotics

Soluble Fiber

Refined Carbohydrates

Psychobiotics

Gut Flora

Micronutrients

Complex Carbohydrates

Match the psychobiotic to how they help the body and mind. Where can you find them?

1. lactobacillus rhamnosus and plantarum

2.Bifidobacterium longum

3. Lactobacillus reuteri

4. Galacto-oligosaccharides (GOS)

- Prevents pathogenic organism growth and has been succesfully used to treat depression.
- Anti-inflammatory properties
- Improves mental health
- Reduces stress and anxiety

(Fallis, 2021)

The digestive system, referred to as the gut and brain are deeply connected. **Psychobiotics** are gut bacteria that influence mood. There are **probiotics** and **prebiotics** that can lead to a healthy gut and a healthy mood.

Where is the small intestine?
Where is the large intestine?

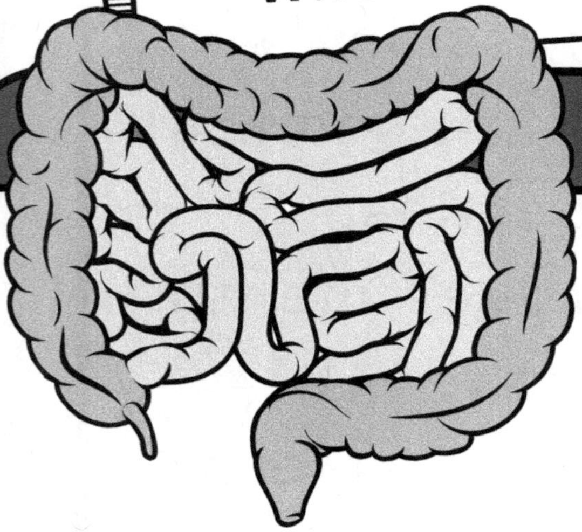

Explain the importance of a healthy gut and how your mood is effected.

List five foods and the prebiotics or probiotics in them and you are willing to eat!

1 ________

2 ________

3 ________

4 ________

5 ________

Research what destroys these good gut bacteria and how to avoid this or bring them back into your gut.

BERRY GOOD *Parfait*

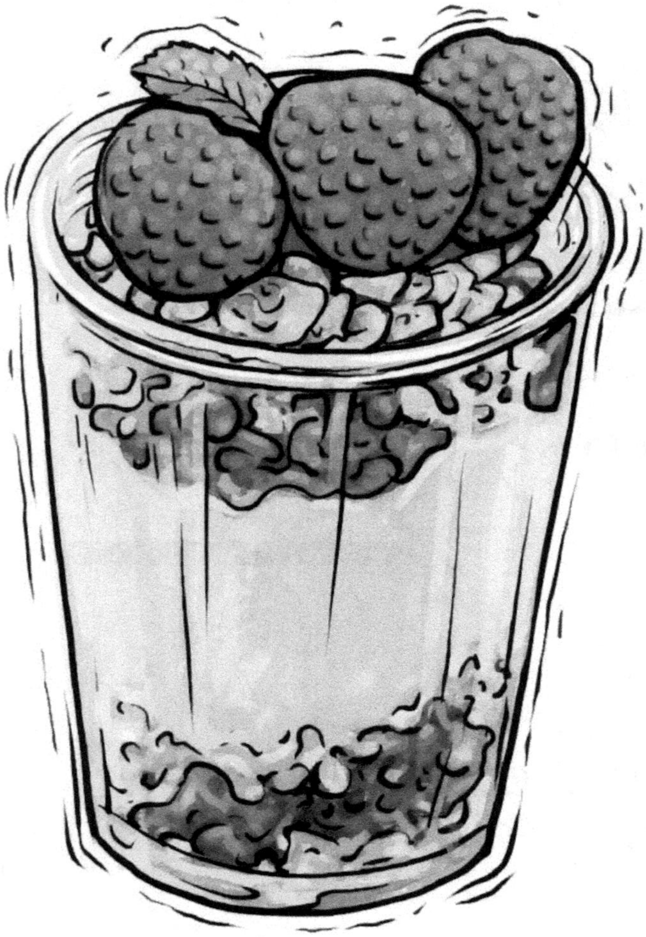

1. Grab a bowl or cup.
2. Make a layer of fruit.
3. Layer with granola.
4. Sprinkle a little ground cinnamon.
5. Make a layer of yogurt.
6. Repeat steps 2-5 until you have the perfect sized parfait.
7. Finish with a layer of granola, fruit to garnish, and lightly drizzle honey over this beautiful parfait.
8. Enjoy!

INGREDIENTS

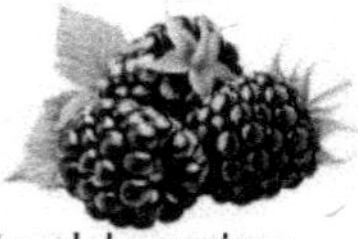
Blackberries

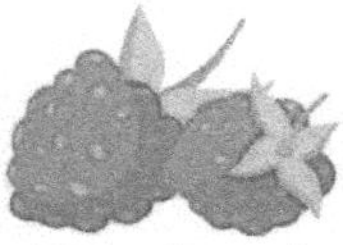
Raspberries

Blueberries

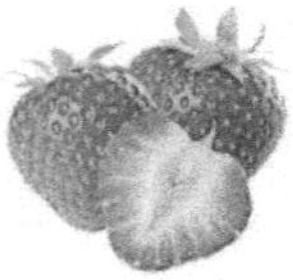
Strawberries

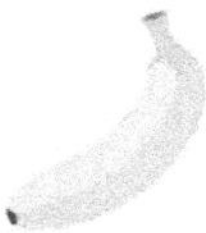
Banana

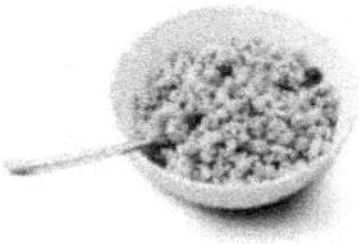
Granola

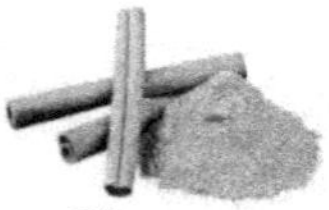
Cinnamon

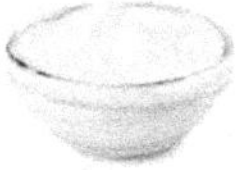
Yogurt

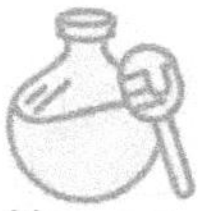
Honey

Parfait Reflection Time

What healthy probiotics do you have in this recipe?

Would you make this recipe different?

What ingredients can be used to make a healthy granola? (pg. 131-132)

Did you use any superfoods or organic foods in this recipe?

How does your mind and body feel after making and eating your parfait?

When can you eat this meal/snack?

To save time, could you make this ahead of time?

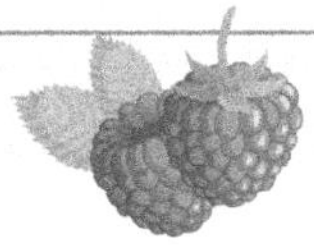

Rewrite your version of the recipe, making changes to quantities, steps, ingredients, or anything else you find fitting.

Recipe Name

Procedure

Yield

Cost

Time

Ingredients

How much would you charge?

What is your profit margin?

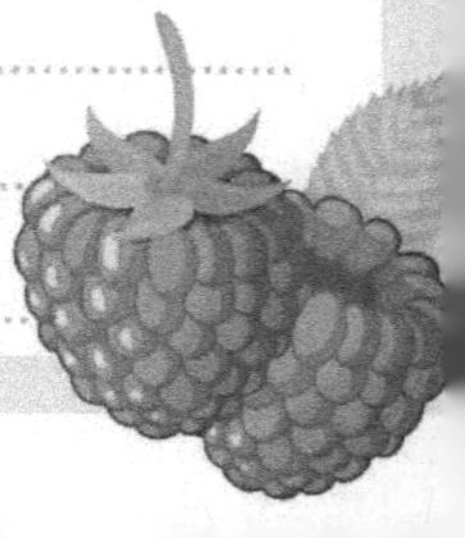

Alkaline Abbey

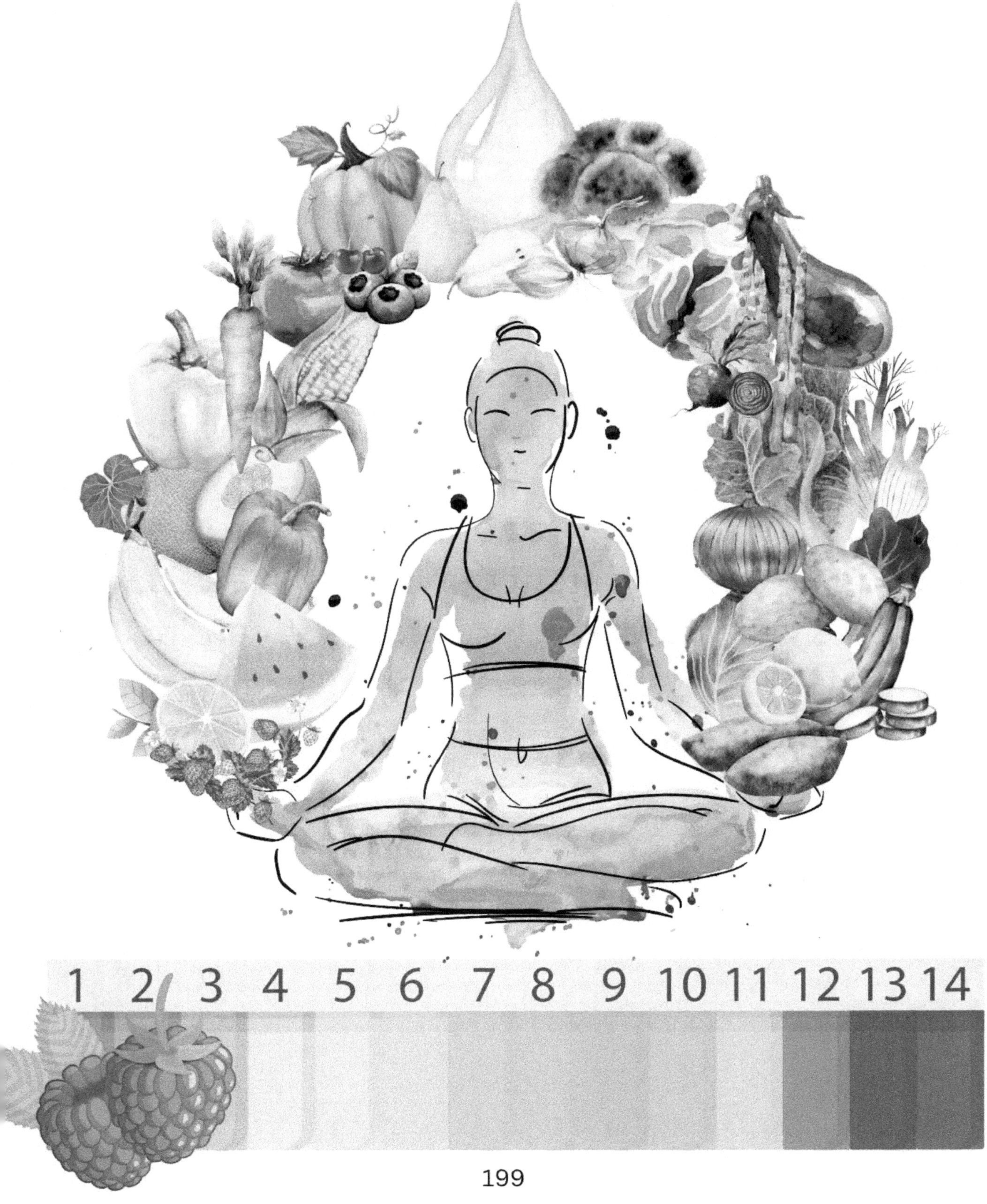

In the Standard American Diet (SAD) of today, the average American is consuming highly processed foods, sugary beverages, meats, dairy products, and are experiencing high amounts of stress. Each of these elements can add up to an overly acidic pH in the body. What does this mean? An overly acidic environment for the body is a common cause of disease and sickness. Some acids in our body are essential, such as in the respiratory and the digestive track. However, too much acid in the body is not good, a healthy balance is key. A few side effects of an unhealthy acidic pH can include agitation, anxiety, shortness of breath, rapid heartbeat, headache, fatigue, and many diseases and cancers. Have you ever experienced any of these symptoms?

How can you avoid these symptoms? These symptoms may not be possible to avoid. However, you can do your part to reduce the likeliness of them being part of your life by eating less acidic foods, more alkaline foods, regular and active exercising, and having a healthy and calm mind and emotions. Each aspect plays a role towards our wellbeing and when we neglect ourselves, our health takes a toll.

How do you know if a food is acidic? A simple way to guess if a food is acidic is to ask yourself a few questions:

- Is this food sweetened with added sugars?
- Are there preservatives?
- Does this food come out of a package?
- Is there dairy or meat in this food?

If you answered yes to any of these questions, most likely the food leans closer to the acidic side of the pH scale. This is not to be feared, but use this knowledge to balance the pH by adding alkaline rich foods to your meal, such as the ones on the next few pages.

Alkaline Foods

Connect the word to the correct drawing.

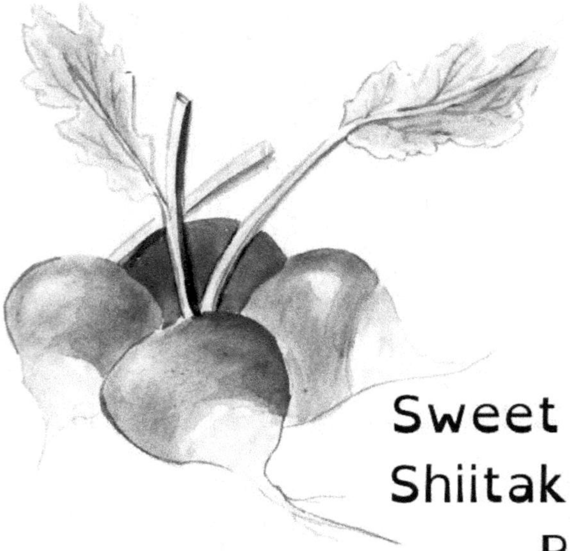

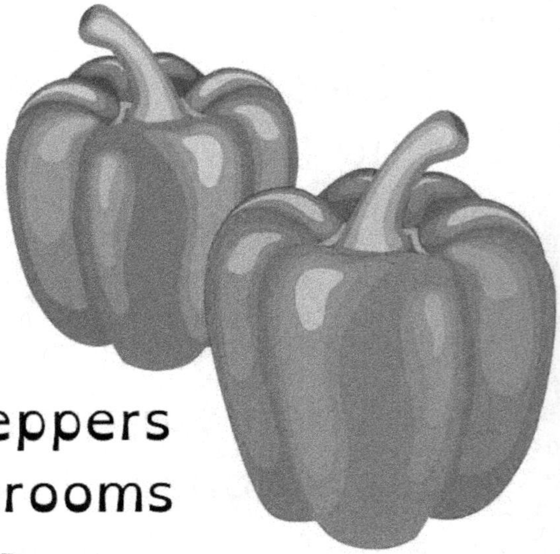

Yams
Sweet Red Peppers
Shiitake Mushrooms
Radishes
Sweet Green Peppers
Russet Potatoes
Shallots
Fennel

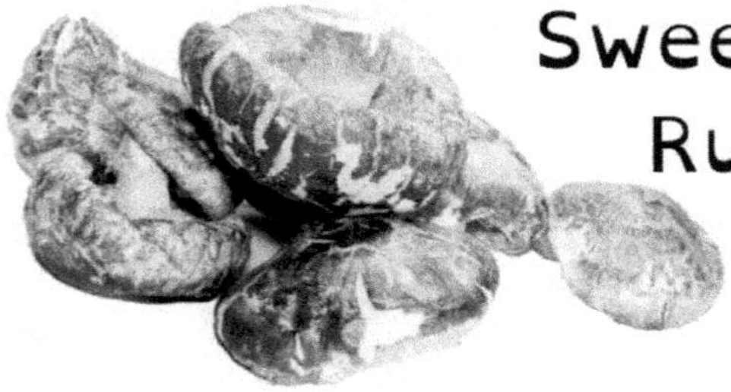

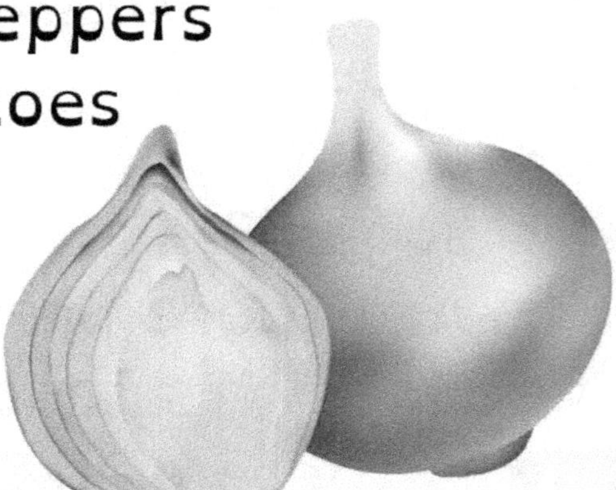

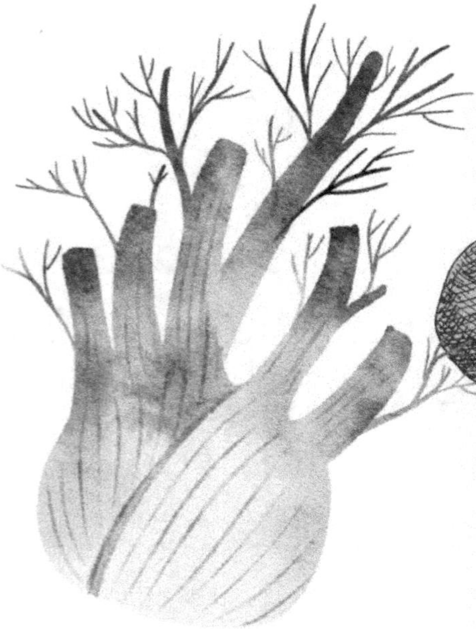

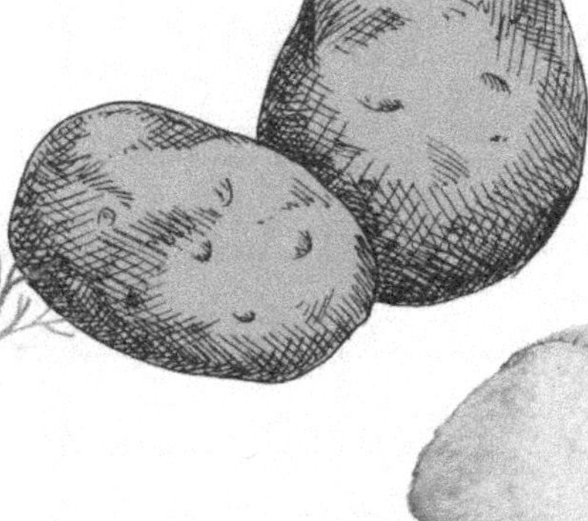

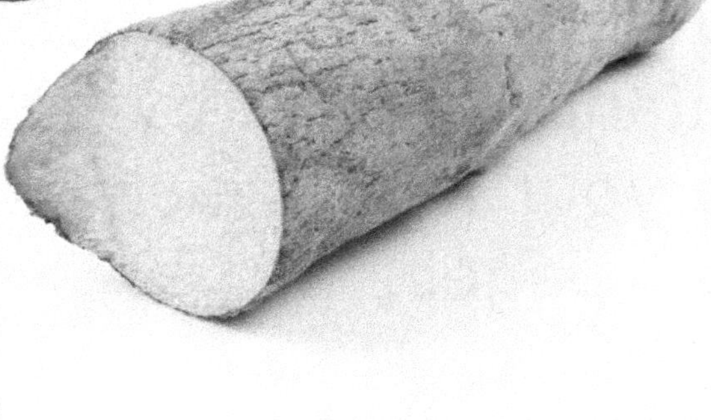

Alkaline Greens

Connect the word to the correct drawing.

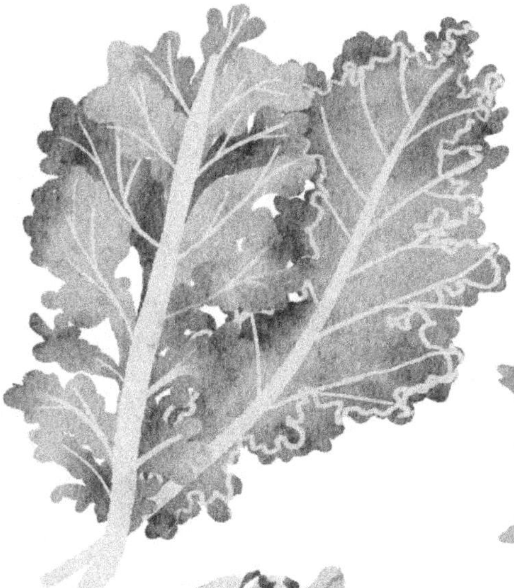

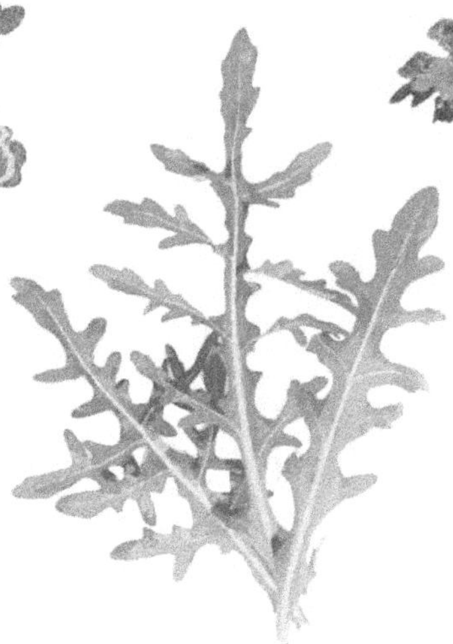

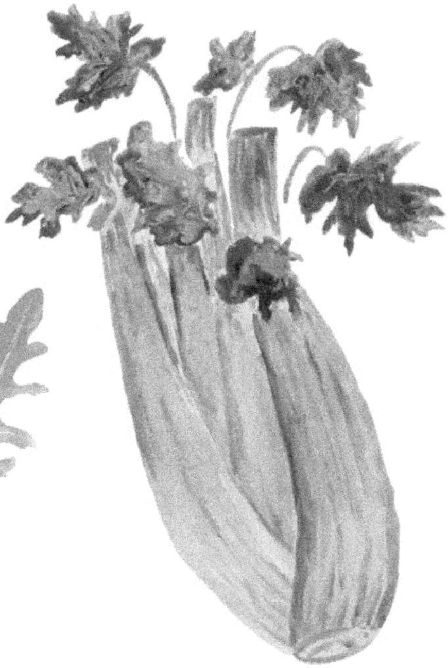

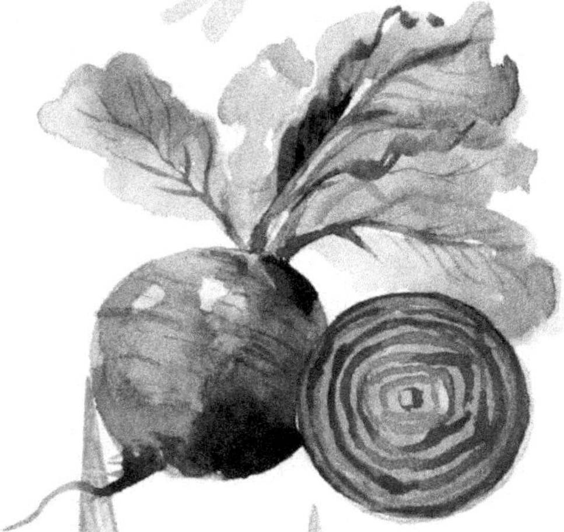

Arugula
Celery
Swiss Chard
Spinach
Kale
Beet Greens
Seaweed

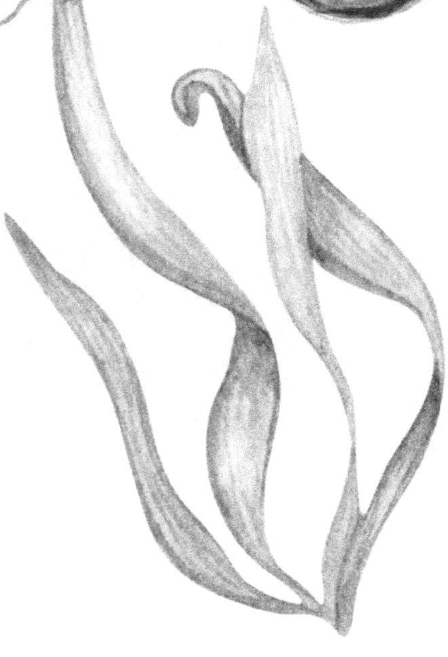

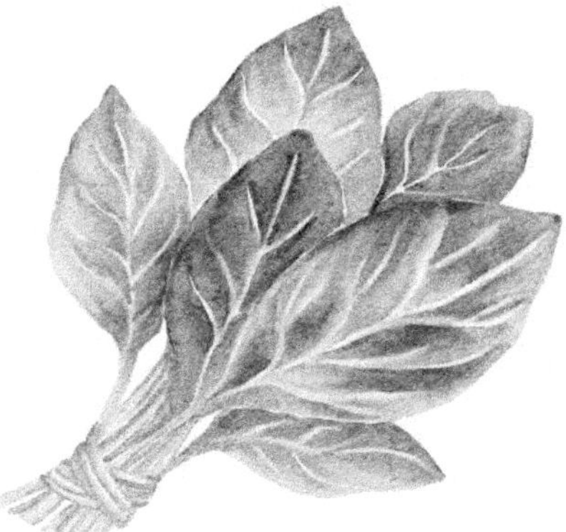

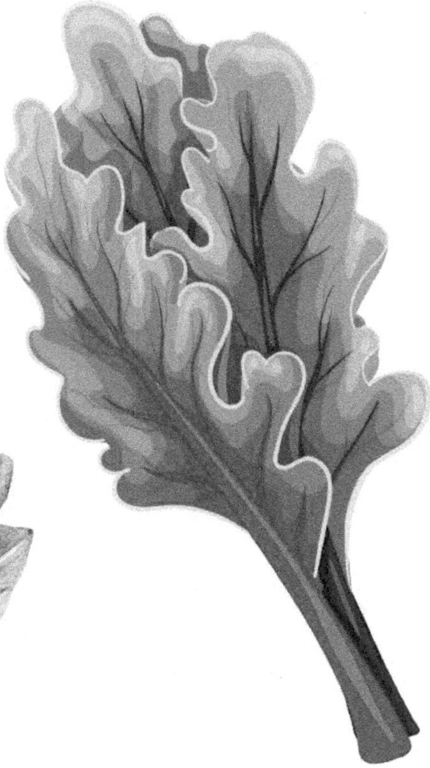

Alkaline Sweets

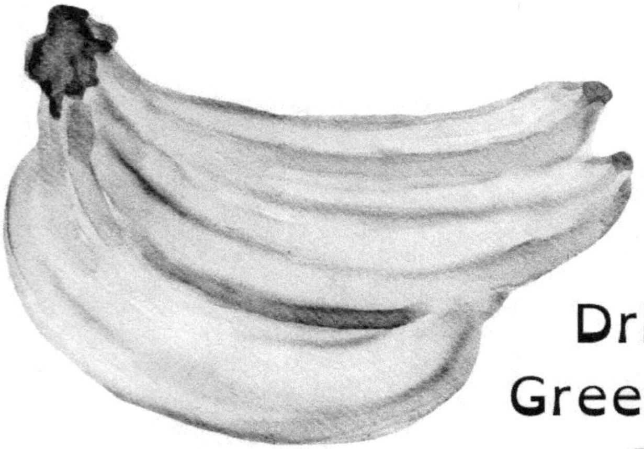

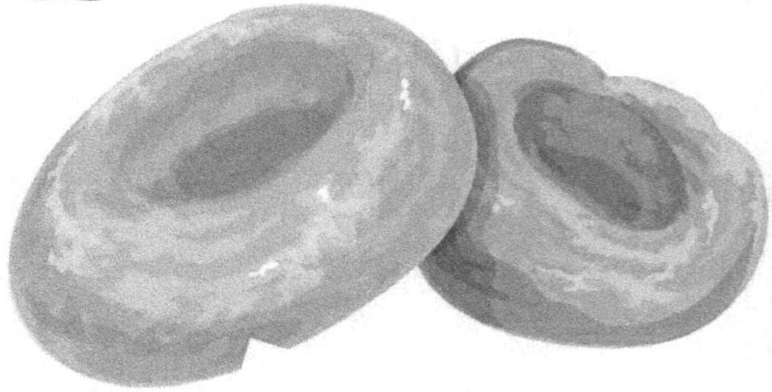

Dried Apples
Greenish Bananas
Molasses
Dried Apricots
Dried Figs
Raisins
Dried Peaches
Medjool Dates

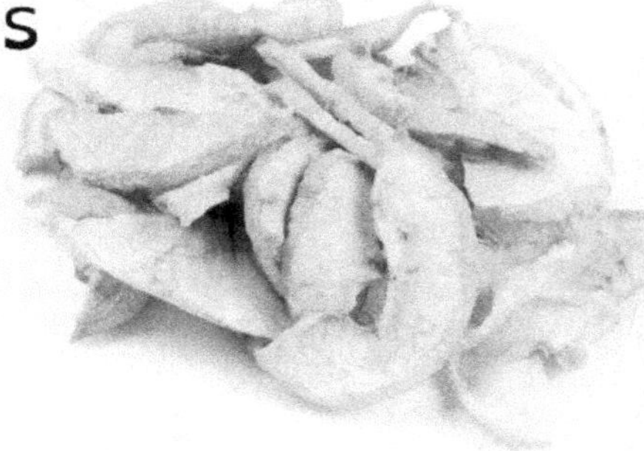

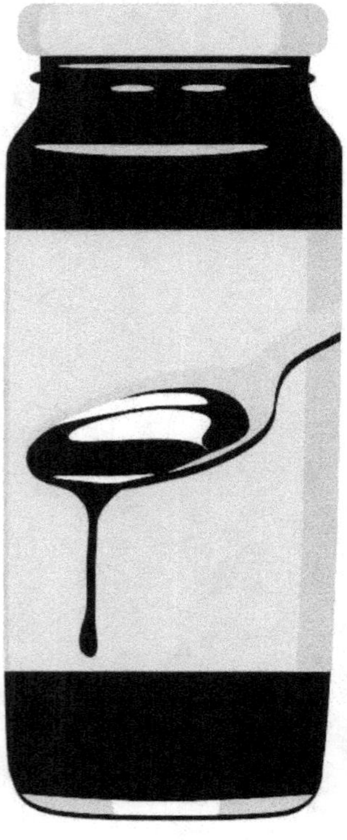

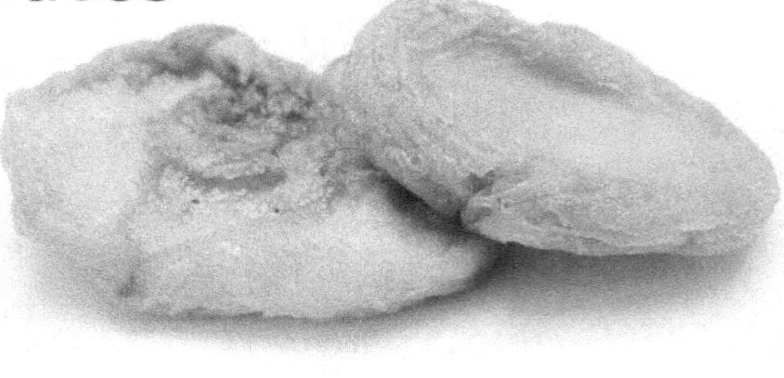

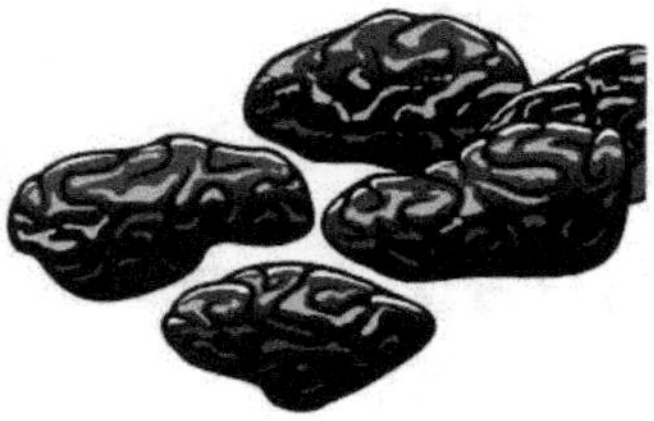

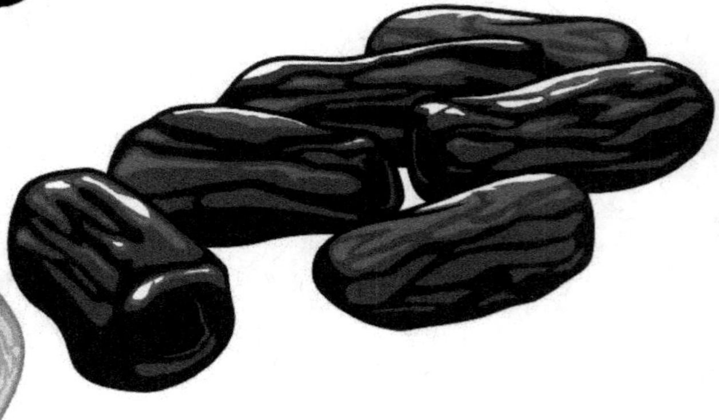

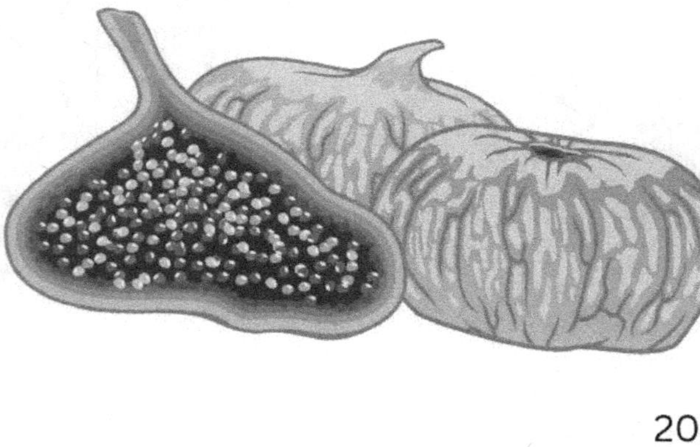

Draw the pH scale. Label the acidic and alkaline sides. Where is water on the scale?

Explain what the PRAL food scale means/stands for and what does it do?

Explain how the numbers relate differently on the PRAL scale than on the pH scale.

If a food has a PRAL score of 47, is this acidic or alkaline?

If a food has a PRAL score of -14, is this acidic or alkaline?

List some of your favorite foods in each category below. Write the PRAL score for each one and label if it is acidic or alkaline.

Meat, Seafood & Dairy:

Fruits & Vegetables:

Grains & Legumes:

Beverages & Desserts:

Explain how you can use the PRAL tool to eat a healthy balanced diet.

Look at some of your favorite foods that have an acidic PRAL score. What food items could you pair them with to balance out the pH?

Be sure to label how you determine your answer. Example: -14 + 21 = 7. Seven is much better than 21 in relation to a healthy PRAL score.

Acid or Alkaline?

Find and highlight the acidic foods below in yellow, orange, or red and highlight the alkaline foods in green or blue.

Raw Cacao	**Cheese**	**Turmeric**	**Flax Meal**	**Mushroom**	**Eggs**
Dried Fruit	**Hot Dogs**	**Cilantro**	**Sour Cherries**	**Lemon**	**Ginger**
Cauliflower	**Pumpkin**	**Croissant**	**Himalayan Salt**	**Garlic**	**Carrots**

O	Y	M	B	N	U	A	C	M	R	T	S	S	F	H
D	T	E	O	H	W	I	P	U	E	L	O	T	L	O
E	E	M	U	I	L	U	N	S	W	A	U	N	A	T
F	E	J	L	A	M	A	Q	H	O	S	R	A	X	D
L	B	J	N	P	G	V	Y	R	L	N	C	S	M	O
K	P	T	K	T	B	Z	Q	O	F	A	H	S	E	G
W	R	I	N	R	T	Y	I	O	I	Y	E	I	A	S
O	N	L	U	K	E	Q	O	M	L	A	R	O	L	N
E	S	E	E	H	C	G	J	J	U	L	R	R	V	A
C	A	R	R	O	T	S	N	L	A	A	I	C	V	C
C	I	R	E	M	R	U	T	I	C	M	E	J	I	U
Y	Q	E	T	C	X	G	Q	A	G	I	S	L	G	T
T	I	U	R	F	D	E	I	R	D	H	R	Z	H	P
T	S	U	J	Q	E	K	B	P	A	A	D	Z	P	N
R	A	W	C	A	C	A	O	P	G	E	G	G	S	V

Balanced Lifestyle

Bringing a healthy pH to your body can be achieved with a great diet, but you need to remember exercise and stress levels play another key role to your health. A few techniques to improve a stressful moment or day can be with positive affirmations, taking calm deep breaths, meditation, quiet time, dancing, fun sports, exercise, and laughter. Describe a situation where you brushed off a not so great mood. What techniques did you use? Research this topic and write your discoveries.

By taking in those calm deep breaths or heavy breathing during exercise, your oxygen levels increases through your blood, clearing away stress (acidic pH). Breathing releases the acidic carbon dioxide in our breath. When we get stressed we tend to hold and shorten our breath, thus holding more carbon dioxide and creating anxiety and acid in our bodies. Breathing slowly and calmly can help our body and mind relax. Try taking a nice big inhale in through your nose, hold a few seconds, and slowly release out. Do this calmly a few times. How do you feel? (This exercise is another way to slow a racing mind, simply by focusing on the in and out breath.)

Another strategy to a healthier pH level and wellbeing, is through sweating. Exercise is a spectacular way to release the built up acidic toxins in our body. When you sweat through exercise our body releases healthy "Feel Good" chemicals into your body, that can melt away stress and aid in increasing your pH to the happy zone! Just remember to stay hydrated with healthy fluids, such as an alkaline forming lemon water. What are some of these "Feel Good" chemicals released during exercise and deep breathing?

Practice your cursive handwriting skills!

There are many fun ways to be healthy and feel great. Be the change from the SAD trend to a joyful, healthy, and vibrant lifestyle. Use the knowledge you have obtained through this book and your research as momentum to live a great and healthy life. By eating nutritious foods found in nature, keeping a positive and peaceful mindset, and having a fun and active exercise program you are on your way to a healthy more alkalized state of being!

HEALTH IS WEALTH

ALKALINE FORMING LEMON *Icey*

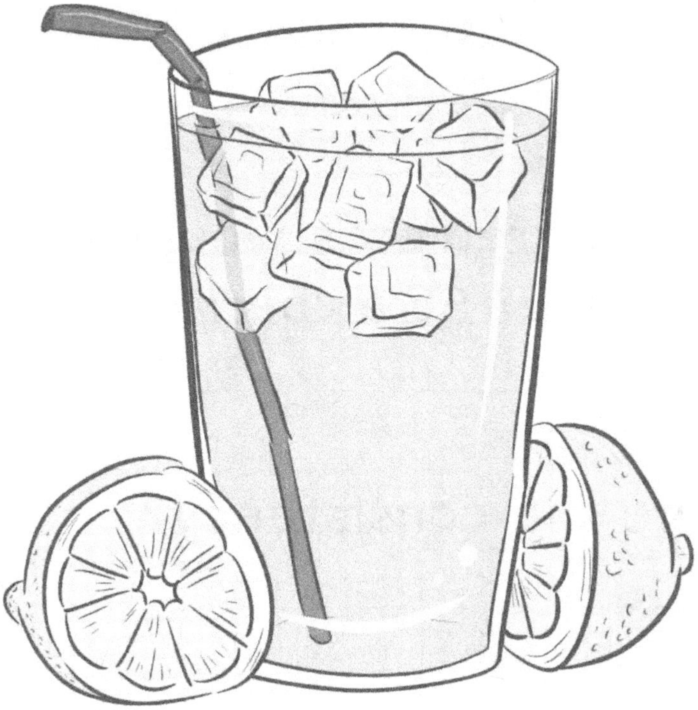

INGREDIENTS

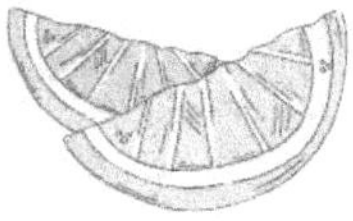

Lemon Juice

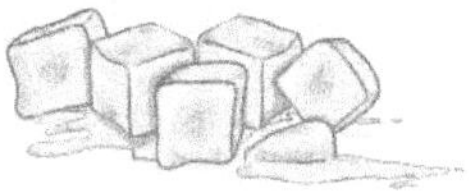

Ice Cubes

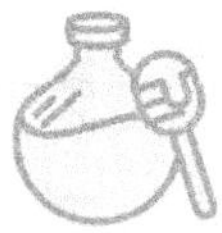

Honey

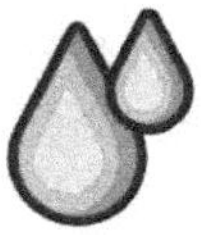

Water

BLEND TOGETHER & ENJOY

½ - 1 Lemon Juiced 1/2 cup Ice Cubes	1-3 Tablespoons Honey 3/4 cup Water

Icey Reflection Time

Did you enjoy this recipe?

Would you consider adding or substituting tea, juice, or another liquid or ice to this recipe?

What other ingredients would you add to this drink? Kale? Strawberries?

Did you like the consistency?

By naming a few health benefits this drink has, how could you describe, advertise, influence, or suggest this healthy drink to others?

How much would you pay for this drink?

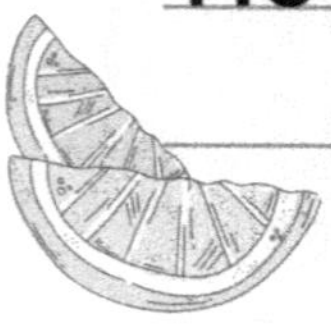

Rewrite your version of the recipe, making changes to quantities, steps, ingredients, or anything else you find fitting.

Recipe Name

Procedure

Yield

Cost

Time

Ingredients

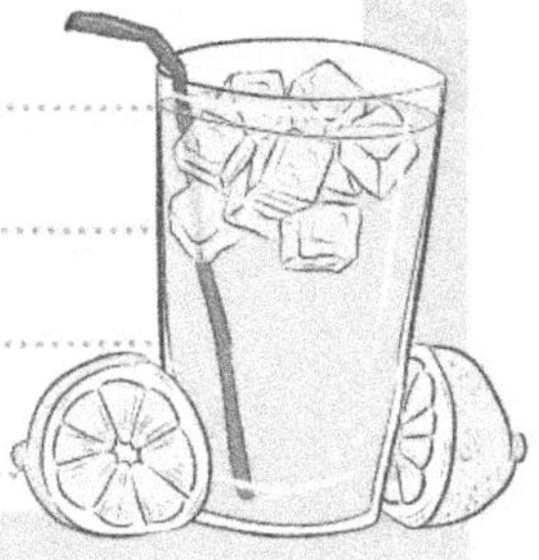

How much would you charge for 16 oz?

What is your profit margin?

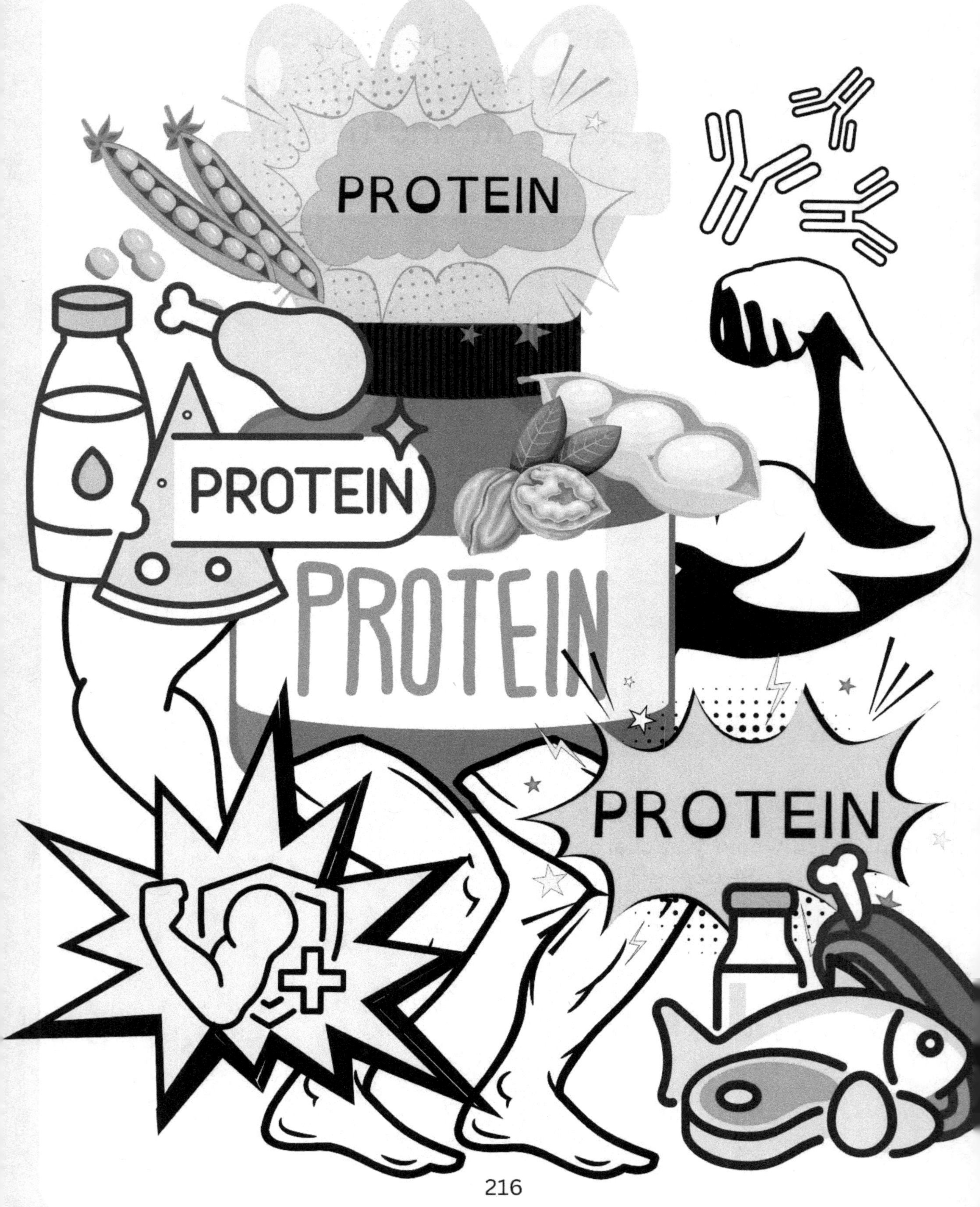
PROTEIN
PROTEIN
PROTEIN
PROTEIN

What is protein?

What types of protein are there?

Where does protein come from?

Are some types of protein better than others?

Describe the importance of proteins in your diet, growth, and health.

List at least 7 foods rich in protein. How much protein do they each have per serving?

Describe a **vegetarian** diet. What protein rich foods can they eat?

Describe a **vegan** diet. What protein rich foods can they eat?

What are complete proteins and how are they important for our bodies? Describe and name some examples.

Name at least 5 complete protein options for a vegetarian, vegan, and 'normal' diet.

How do **amino acids** relate to protein?

How do amino acids help the body?

List at least 7 foods rich in amino acids. Are any of them superfoods?

The 9 Essential Amino Acids Are:

Our bodies do not produce these!

List and explain these essential amino acids.

1.

2.

3.

4.

5.

6.

7.

8.

9.

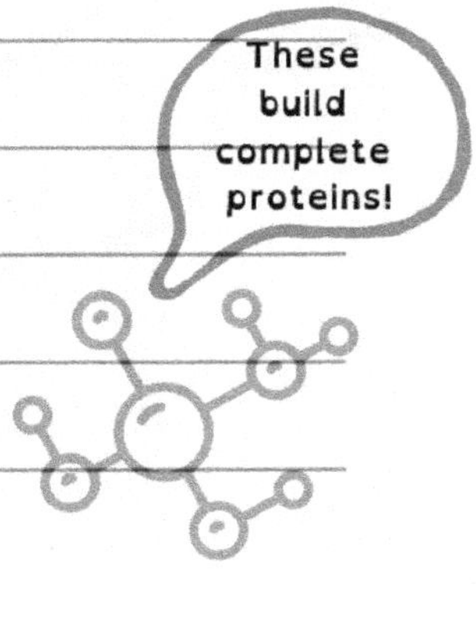

Serving Protein

Write how much protein per serving each food item has.

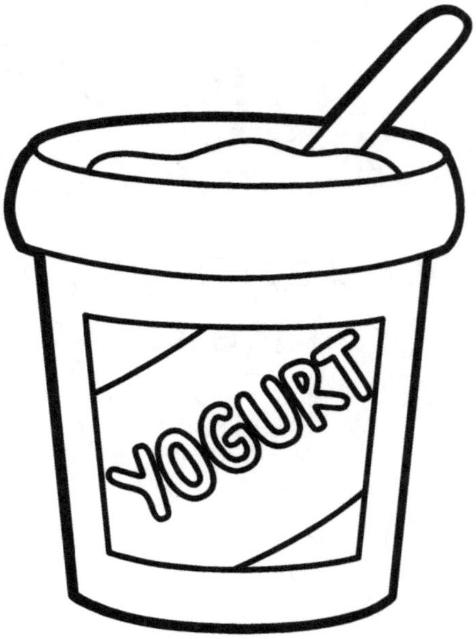

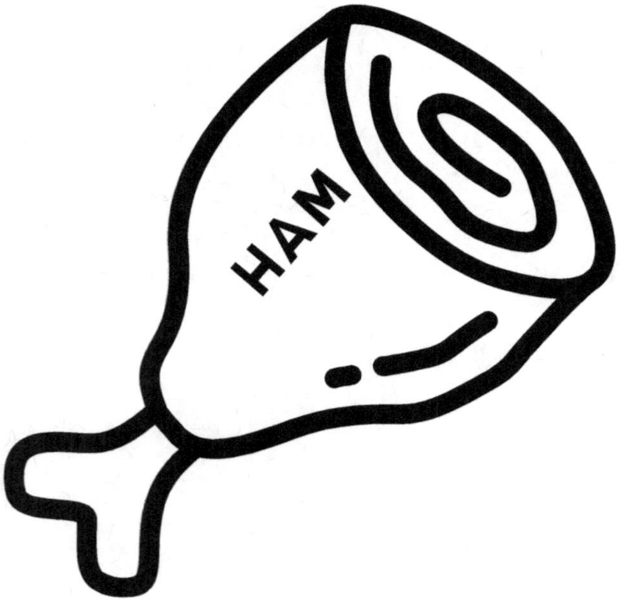

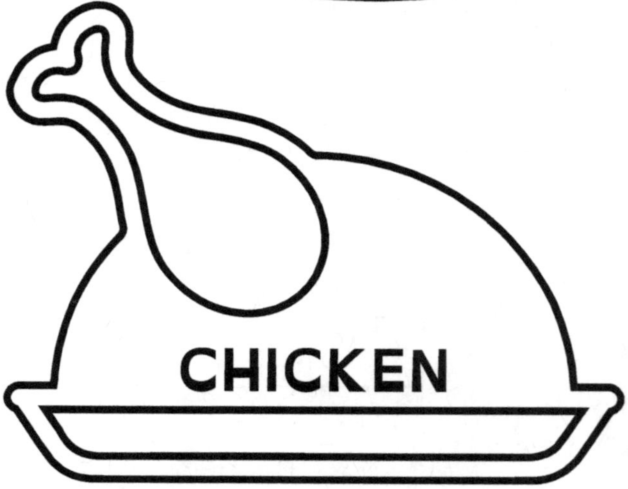

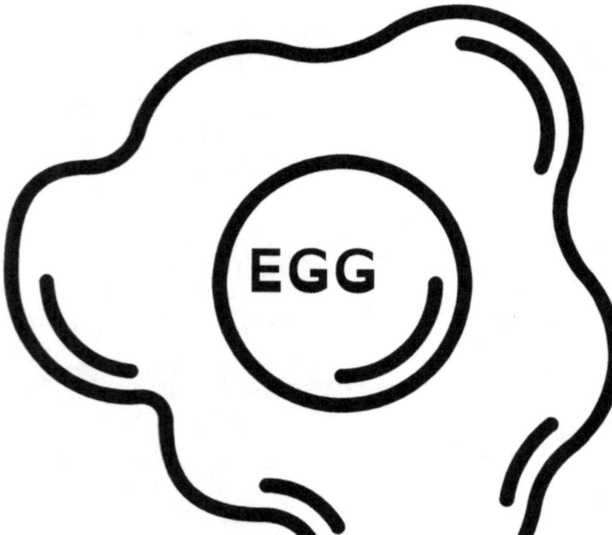

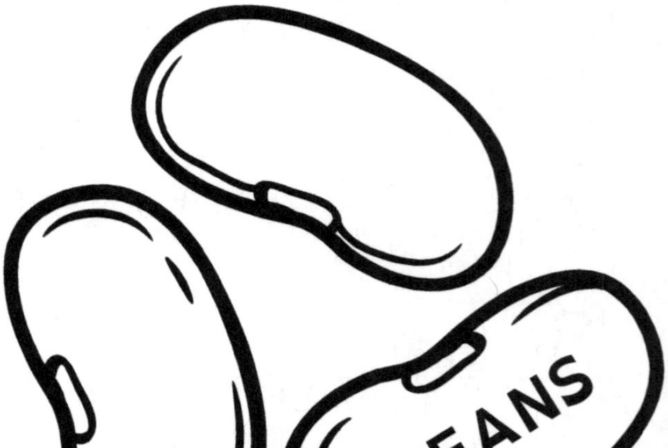

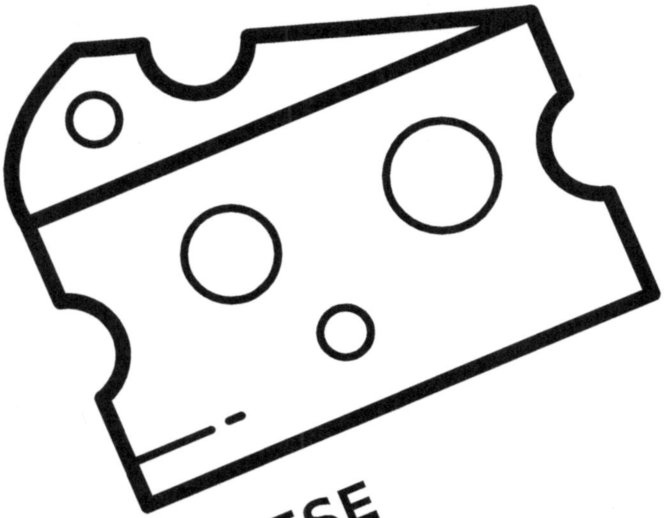

CHEESE

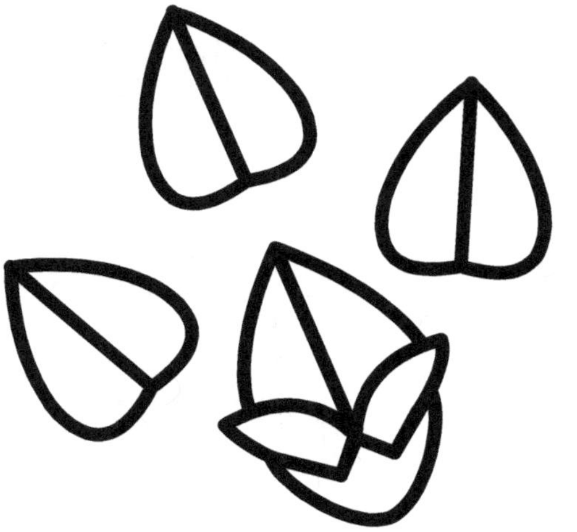

BUCKWHEAT

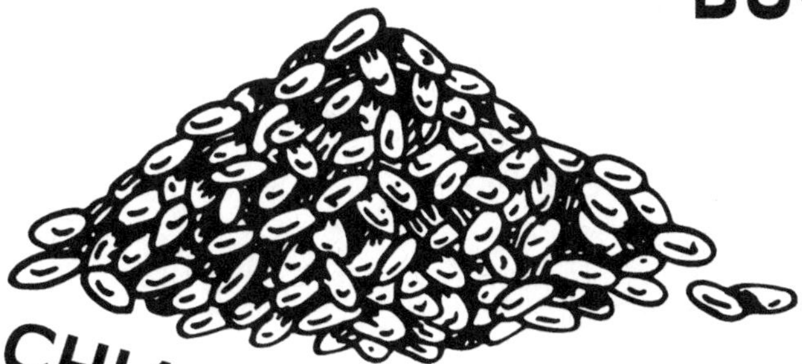

CHIA SEEDS

CHICKPEAS

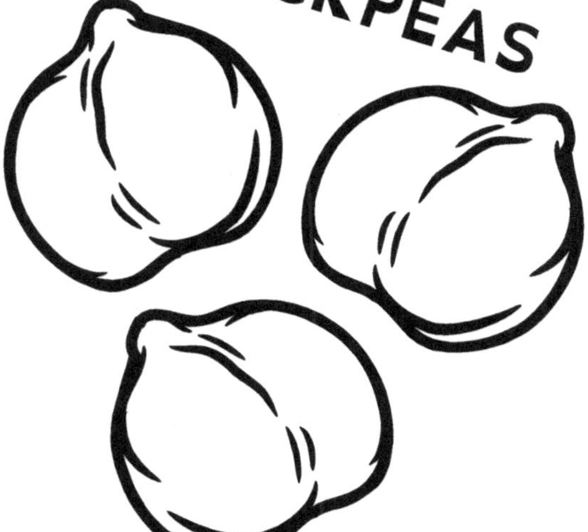

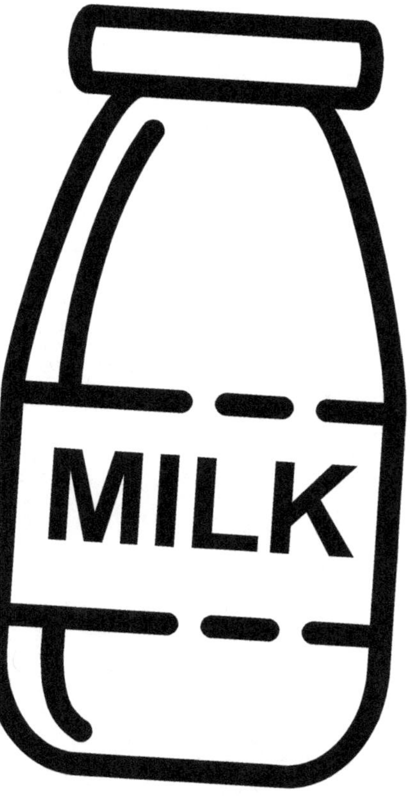

How much protein a day is recommended for a healthy diet?

Are some protein and other food combinations better to have together? Name a few examples.

Name some of your favorite sources of protein.

Make a list of meals, appetizers, drinks, and even deserts that are rich protein. Try to optimize nutrition with the healthiest food combinations.

Practice your cursive handwriting skills!

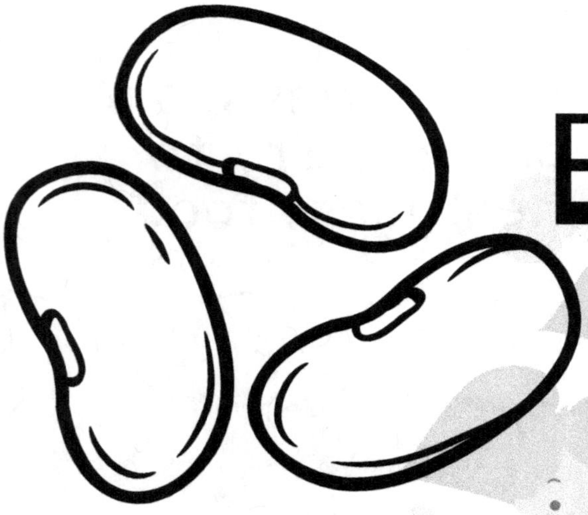

Beans...

Beans...

The Magical Fruit...

The More You Eat...

The More You

!

____

What is the difference between beans and legumes? How are they similar?

List 10 beans or legumes, write the amount of protein, fiber, and fat content per serving and any special nutritional properties.

Connect each bean with the matching picture.

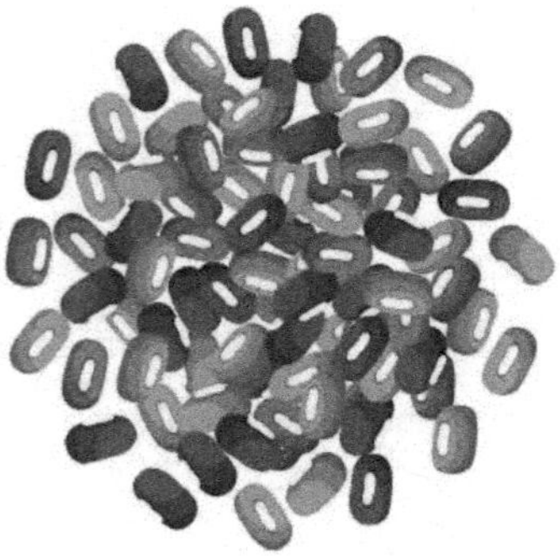

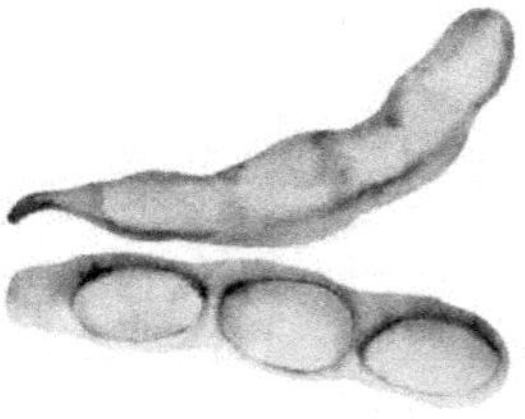

Garbanzo Beans

Lentils

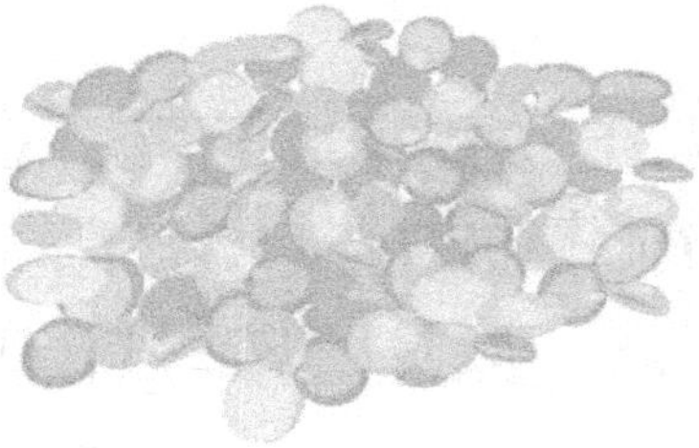

Black Beans

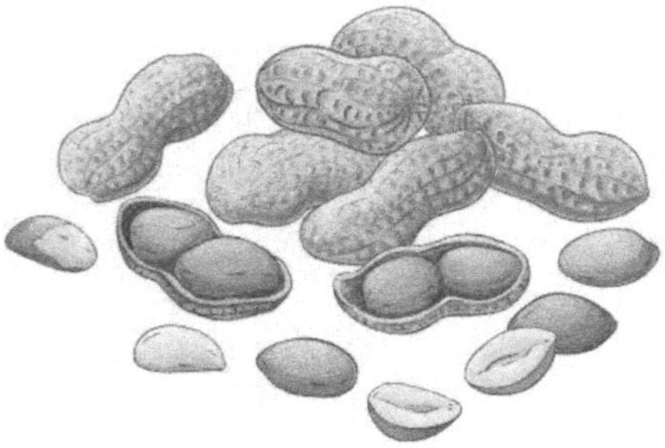

Peas

Soy Beans

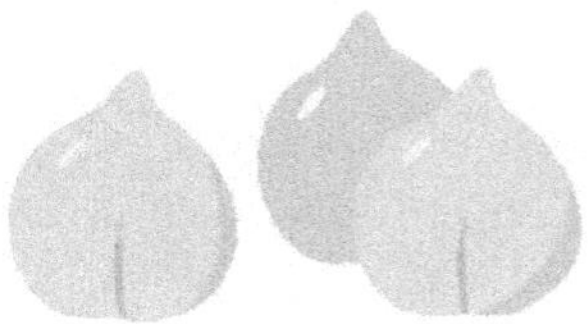

Black-Eyed Peas

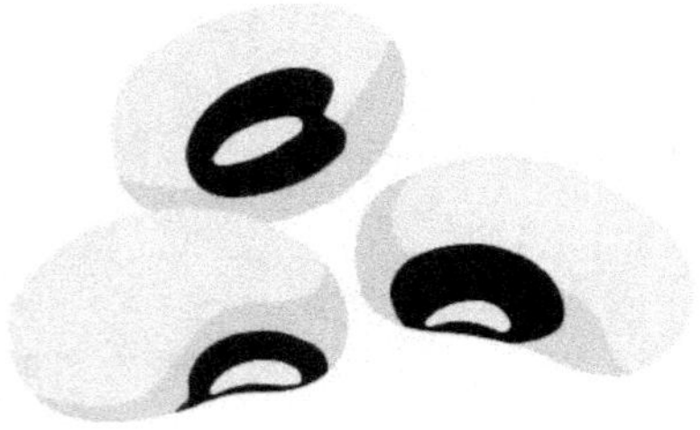

Edamame

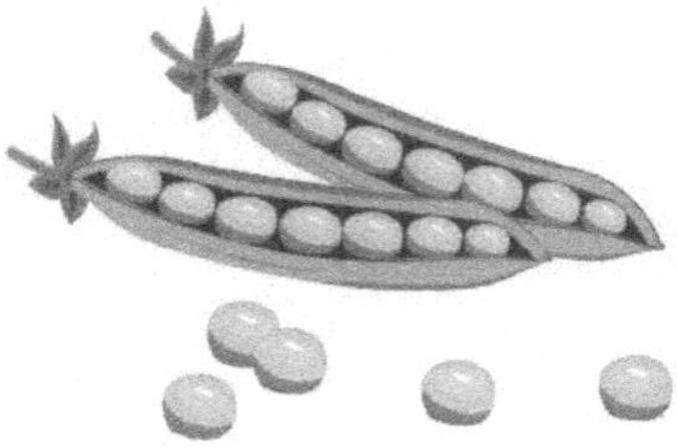

Adzuki Beans

Peanuts

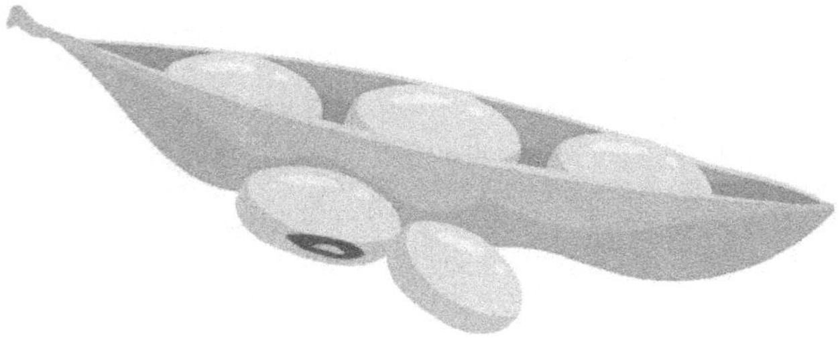

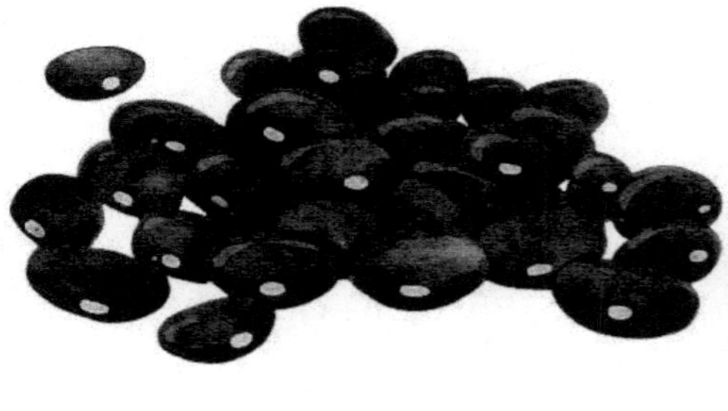

How can vegetarians and vegans use beans and legumes in their diet?

What do beans or legumes need to be paired with to make a complete protein?

Name more healthy combinations.

What are some of your favorite dishes with beans in them?

Are beans and legumes categorized as a carbohydrate or protein? Explain.

Are beans and legumes rich in fiber?

Describe the different types of fiber.

Explain the importance of fiber in a diet and how this effects our body and mind.

Name a few fiber rich foods. Label how much fiber they have per serving.

Nutty Benefits

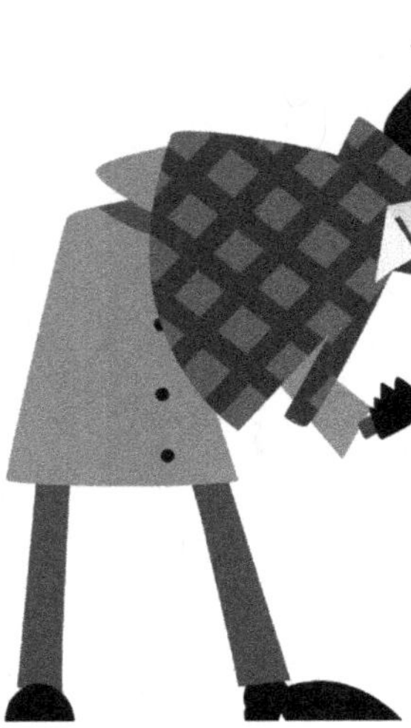

Nuts are often overlooked as a healthy food. Do some investigating and research to uncover what makes these nuts so nutritious. Write your discoveries. List how much protein and fat they have. Be sure to mention the positive benefits of the healthy fats.

Brazilian Nuts

Hazelnuts

Chestnuts

Macadamia Nuts

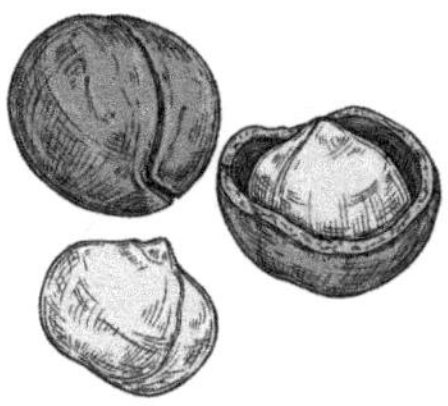

Nutty Ideas

List at least 2 things you can make with each nut. List how much protein and fat each nut has.

Pecans

Walnuts

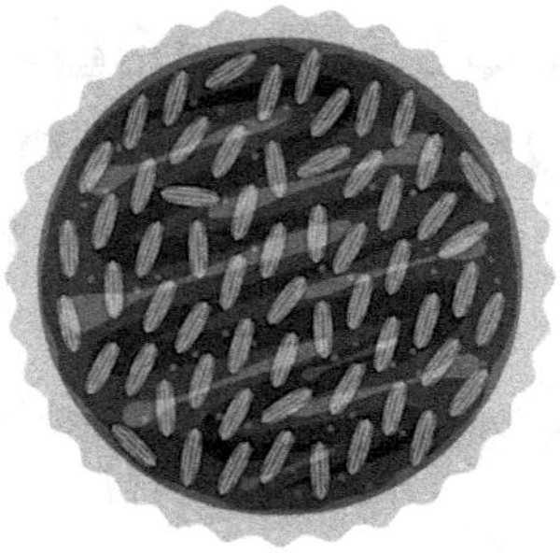

Pistachios

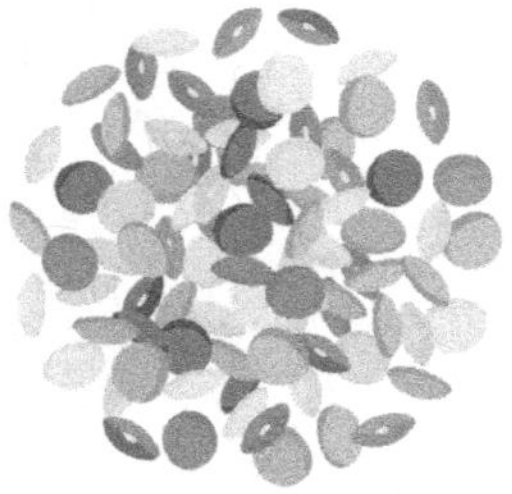

Cashews

Brazilian Nuts

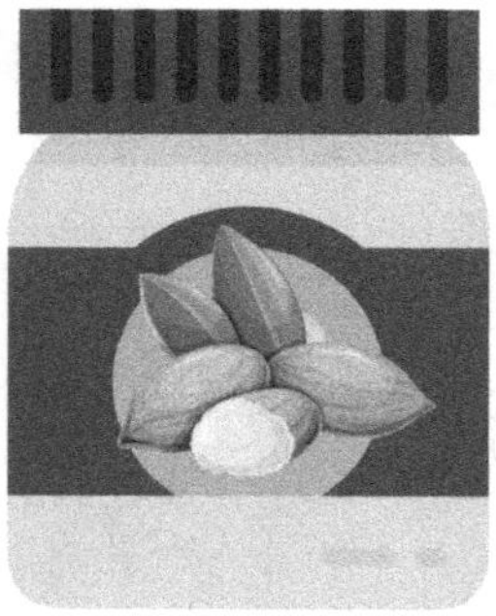

Almonds

Nutty Trivia

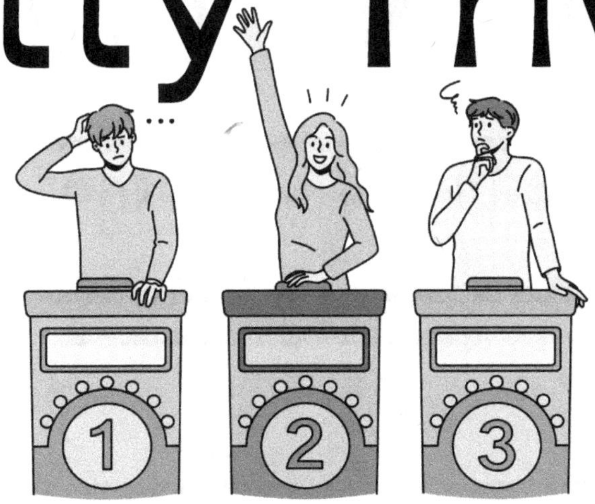

True or False.

Label if you think the statement is true or false, then research to see if you got the correct answers. Use the space to correct the false statements.

Coconuts are considered to be in the nut family.
Cashews are toxic because they are relatives of poison ivy.

Nutty Trivia

Almonds need bees and other pollinators to pollinate.

Peanuts are not a nut because they grow above ground, like other legumes.

Walnuts are the oldest known tree food, dating back to 7,000 BC.

Pistachios are called the "happy nut" in South America.

NUTTY Smoothie

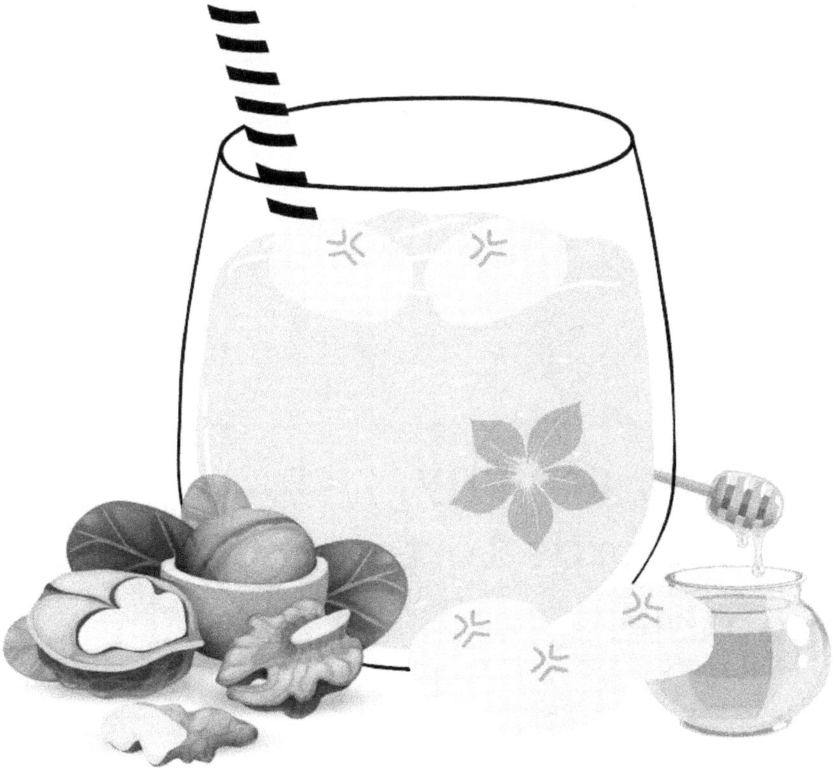

INGREDIENTS

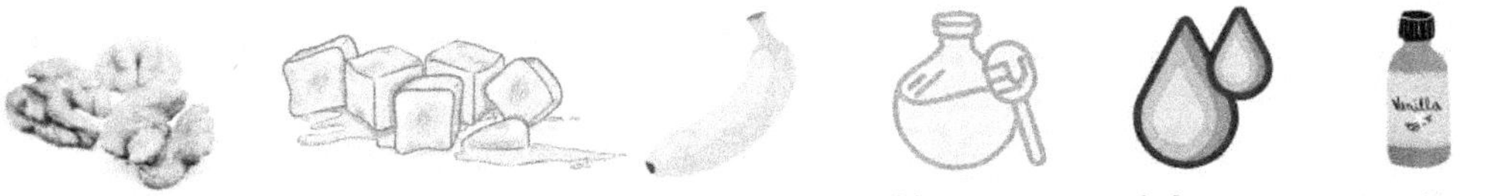

Walnuts | Ice Cubes | Banana | Honey | Water | Vanilla

BLEND TOGETHER & ENJOY

1/3 cup Walnuts or other nut 1/2 cup Ice Cubes 1 Banana, peeled & frozen	1 Tablespoon Honey 1 1/2 cups Water or Milk 1/4 teaspoon Vanilla

Nutty Reflection Time

How much protein is in this smoothie?

Would you like to add yogurt, use a different nut, or add other ingredients to this recipe?

Was it sweet, creamy, rich... use other descriptive words to tell someone about your smoothie.

By naming a few health benefits this drink has, how could you describe, advertise, influence, or suggest this healthy drink to others?

Rewrite your version of the recipe, making changes to quantities, steps, ingredients, or anything else you find fitting.

Recipe Name

Procedure

Yield

Cost

Time

Ingredients

How much would you charge for 16 oz?

What is your profit margin?

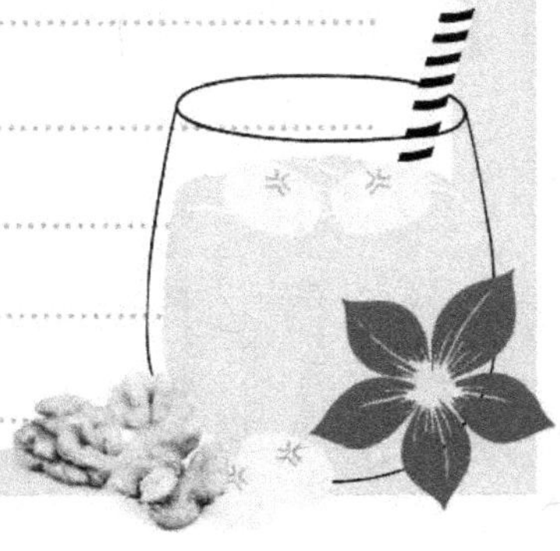

Underwater Food

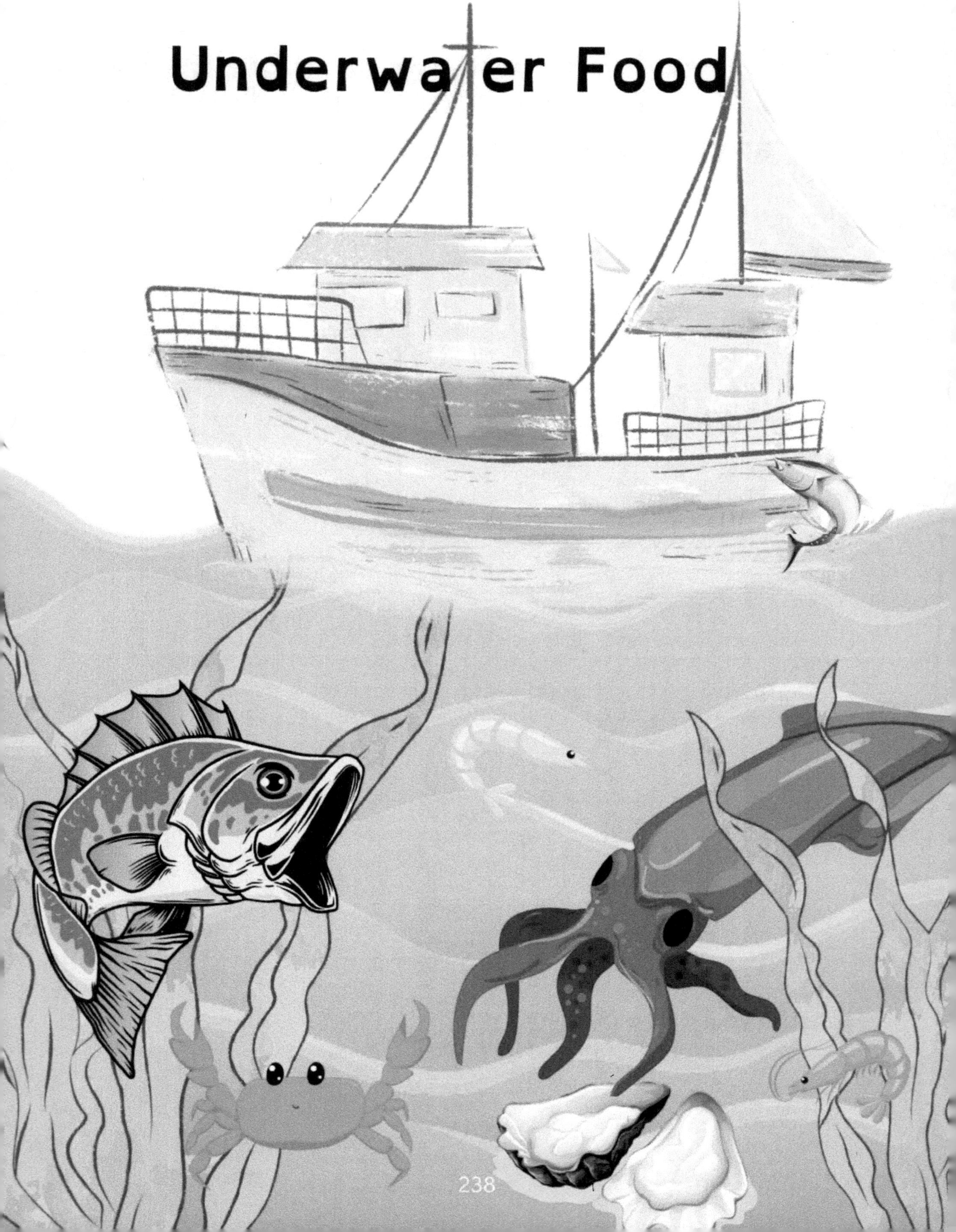

Seafood is very rich in protein. Name some other healthy characteristics and properties of seafood.

What amounts of seafood are recommended?

When you shop in the market or grocery stores, where does the seafood come from?

How are shrimp/prawns commercially grown and harvested?

What about salmon?

Gone Fishing!

Draw what you caught. List the amount of protein and fat per serving.

Shrimp

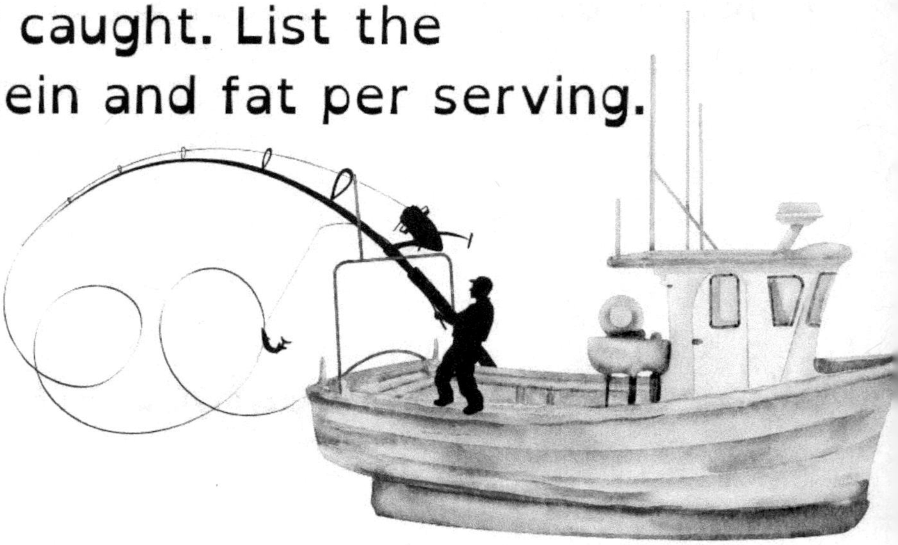

Tuna

Grouper

Flounder

Catfish

Swordfish

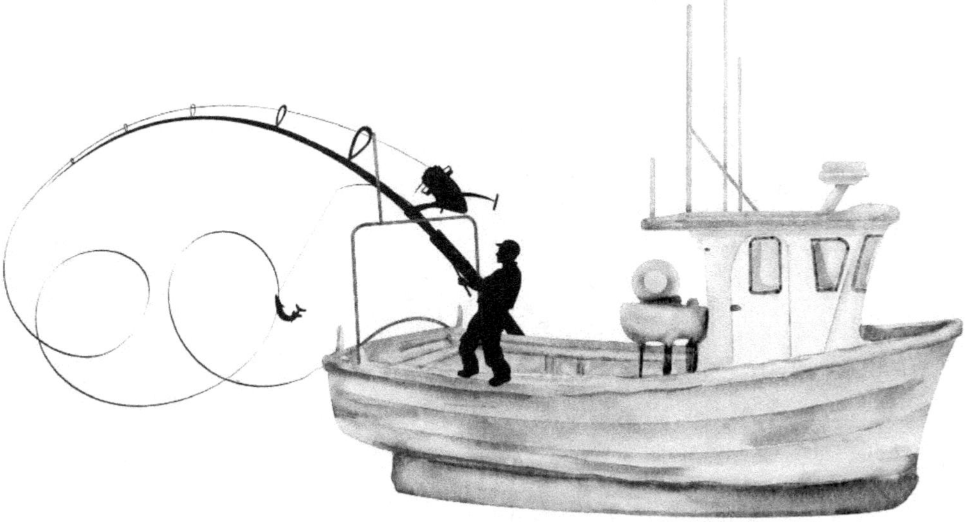

Cod

Mahi-Mahi

Rainbow Trout

Salmon

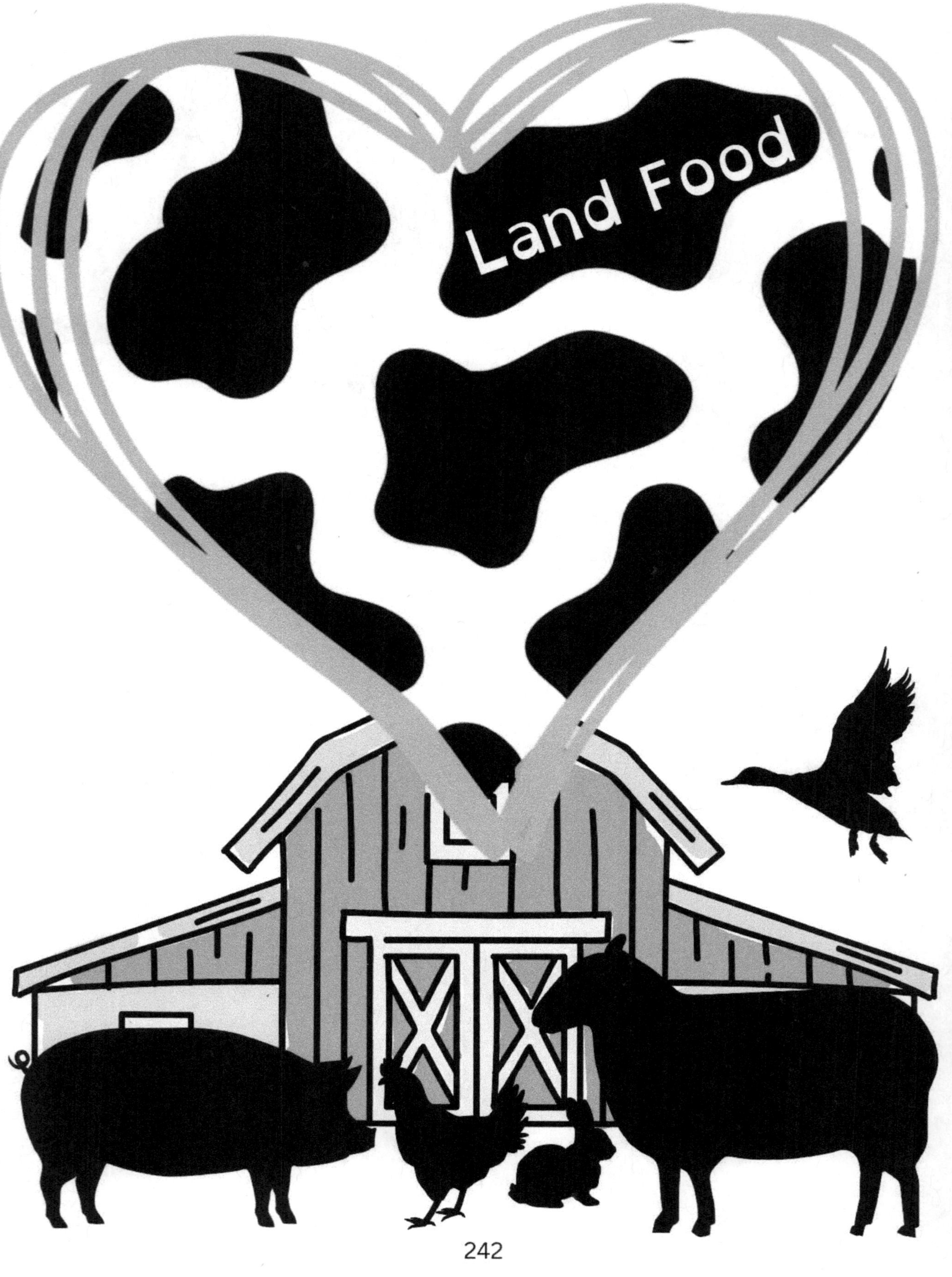
Land Food

What land animals are raised to eat?

When in history were animals first consumed? Why? Explain all that was used of the animal.

Is eating animal meat important in our diet? Explain.

Are lean cuts of meat better? Explain.

Besides protein, what other health benefits can animal meat provide?

Practice your cursive handwriting skills!

Is all meat created equal? Does the farming practices, standards, and animal care impact the quality and taste of meat?

What alternatives would a vegetarian or vegan use instead of meat for their protein and nutrients?

Chicken

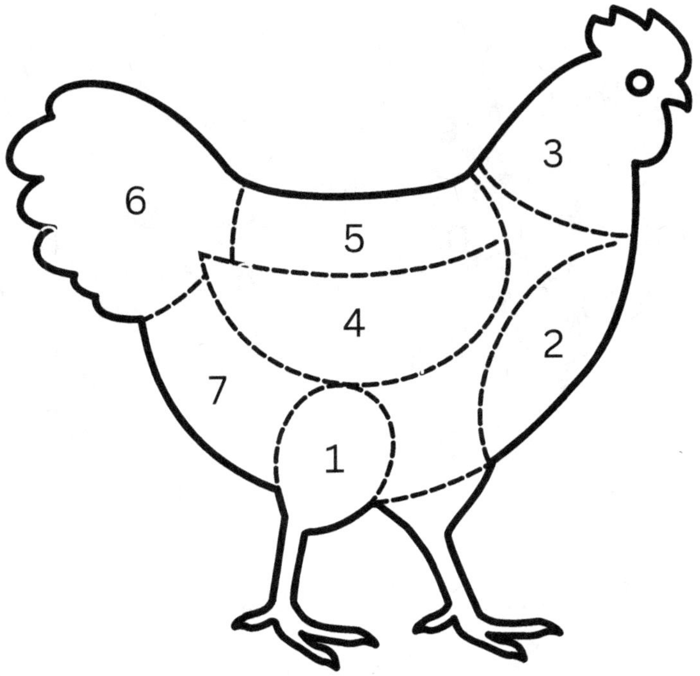

Locate the following cuts of meat and include the fat and protein content:

Tail

Back

Neck

Drumstick

Thigh

Breast

Wing

Pork

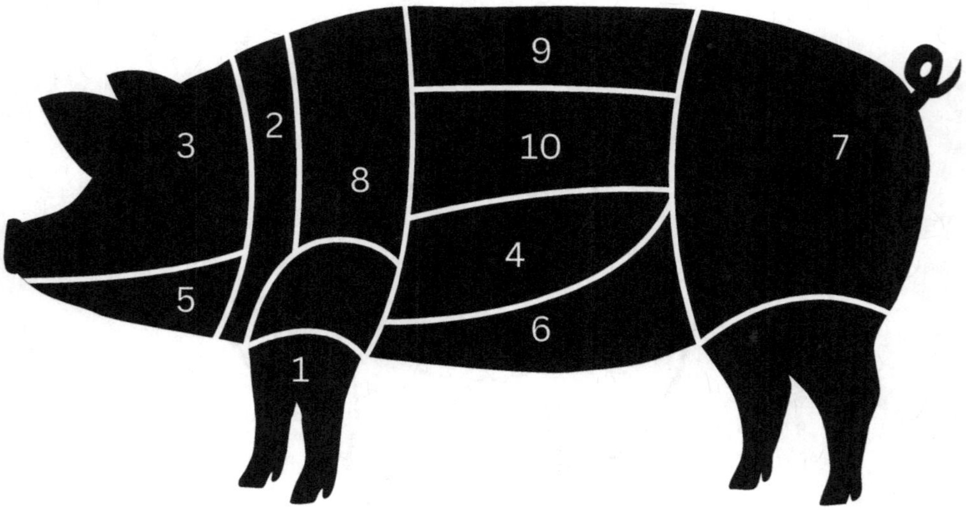

Locate the following cuts of meat and include the fat and protein content:

Jowl
Ham
Hocks and Feet
Back Fat
Head
Spare Ribs
Picnic Ham
Loin
Pork Belly
Pork Shoulder

Where is the bacon?

Beef

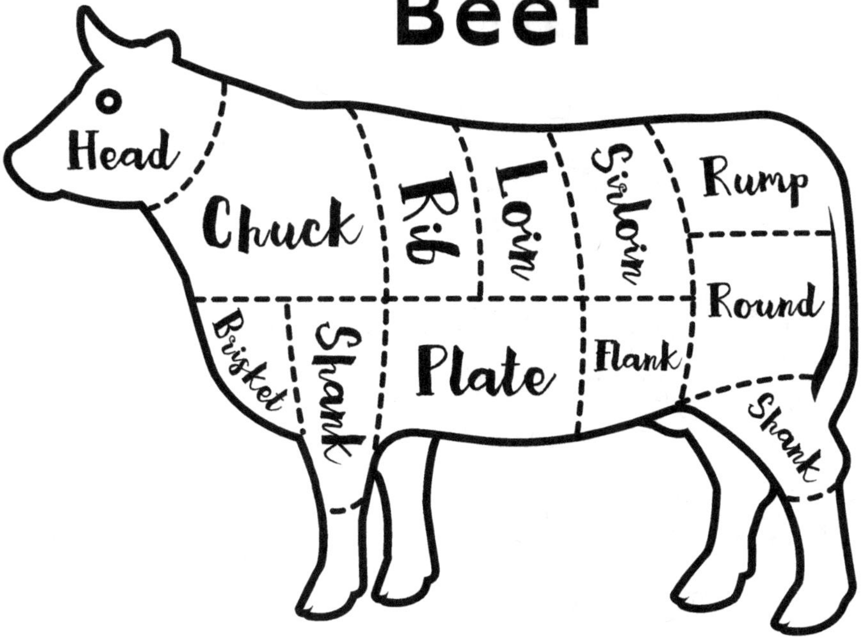

Describe each cut, be sure to include texture, flavor, fat, and protein content.

Protein Math

- Using all the previous pages for help, answer the questions on the next few pages.
- Use the space on each page to show how you got your answer.
- Be sure to include additional foods, remembering to write the amount of protein per serving.
- Use the PRAL scale tool to keep the pH of the meals from getting too acidic, meat and dairy tend to be acidic foods.

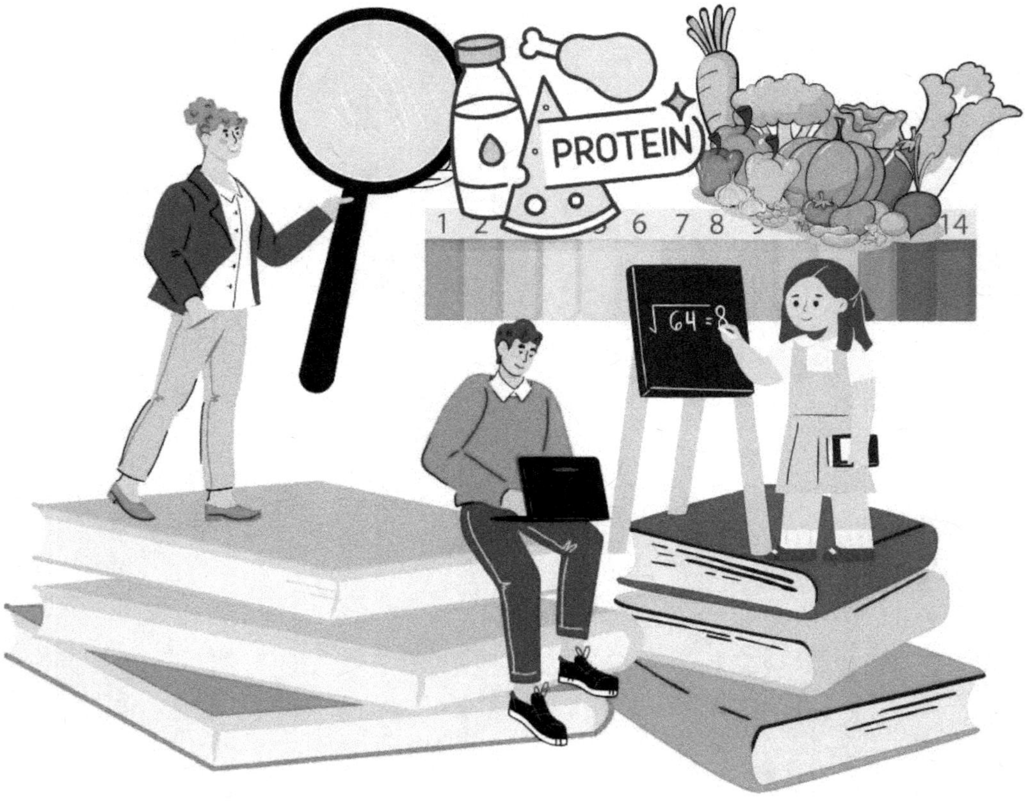

Carly weighs 113 pounds. How many grams of protein are recommended for her daily average?

First, find the recommended protein amount is per pound, then multiply from there.

Carly is trying to increase her daily protein intake by 25%. How much protein will she need to add to her diet? What would her total protein intake be?

Write out a meal plan that includes her new protein needs. Use this space for serving size calculations and notes. Write the meal plan on the next page. Include the PRAL score.

The Protein Meal Plan

Breakfast

Snacks & Sides

Lunch

Snacks & Sides

Dinner

Snacks & Sides

Protein Notes

Doug weighs 190 pounds. He is trying to increase his daily protein intake by 40%. How much protein will he need to eat? Make a food plan for Doug. Include the PRAL score.

The Protein Meal Plan

Breakfast

Snacks & Sides

Lunch

Snacks & Sides

Dinner

Snacks & Sides

Protein Notes

Got Muscle?

Now that you know more about protein, does it really build muscle? Explain.

Why is muscle so important for your body? Explain the benefits and purpose of muscles.

What are a few ways to build muscle?

Meal Planning for You!

Use your knowledge about protein, muscles, healthy food, good mood, and a balanced nutritional pH to apply to yourself.

You weigh ______ pounds. How much protein do you need to eat? Do you want to increase your daily protein intake? Make a food plan for yourself.

Remember to include healthy fats, grains, fiber, fruits, veggies, dairy, fluids, superfoods, and PRAL scores!

Your Healthy Meal Plan

Breakfast

Snacks & Sides

Lunch

Snacks & Sides

Dinner

Snacks & Sides

Health Notes

Drink Up!

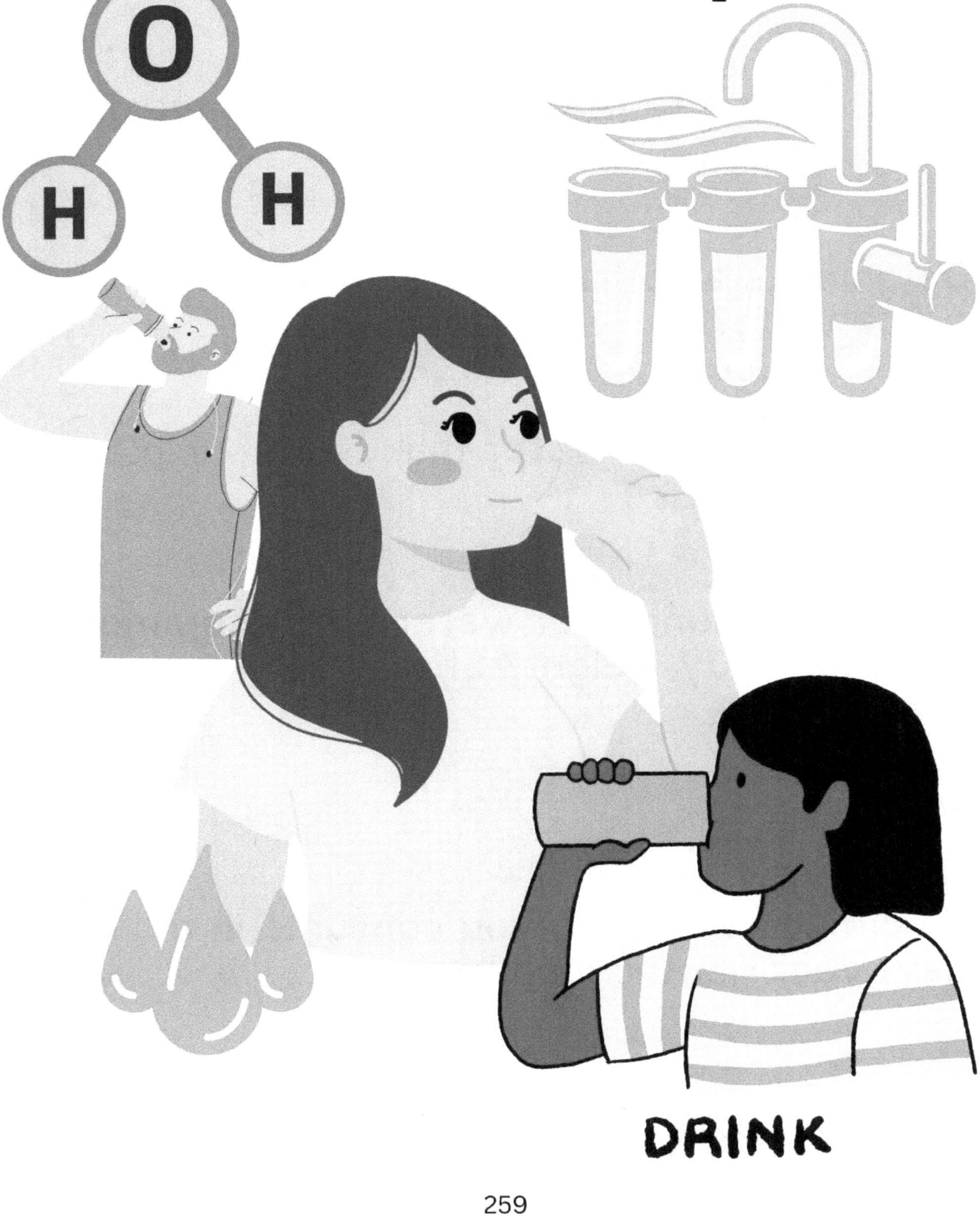

What percentage of water makes up the body?

Is this percentage the same for all ages?

Do animals also have the same water percentage?

What percent of water makes up our planet?

How many ounces of water are recommended for your body weight? Show how you got your answer.

How much water do you consume in a day/week? Is this enough?

What is body dehydration? How does this effect your mind?

List some signs of dehydration.

How can you avoid dehydration?

What is an easy way can you carry water with you where you go?

What types of water containers are healthy options?

Water and Sound Science

Dr. Masaru Emoto studied water. He found water has memory and reacts to its environment. Research Dr. Emoto and his studies on water. Write down some interesting facts that you find.

Name some positive affirmations, uplifting words and phrases.

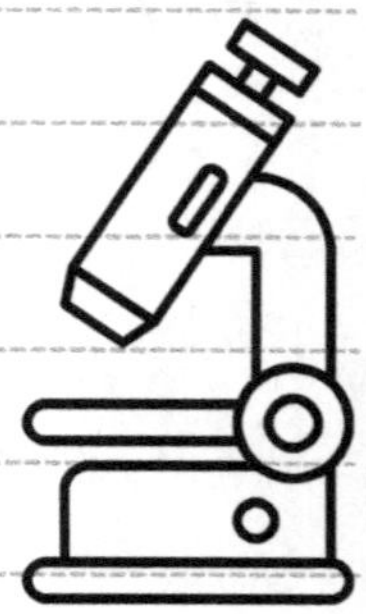

Continue researching Dr. Emoto's studies to complete the next pages.

Draw how water reacted to Bach's **"Air for the G String"** song.

Draw how the water reacted to **heavy metal** music.

What changes do you see in the water from Bach to heavy metal? Why do you think there are these changes?

Draw how the water reacted with the words written in Japanese "**Thank You**" on the bottle.

Draw how the water reacted with the words written in Japanese "**You Fool**" on the bottle.

Describe the changes you see. Why do you think there are these changes?

Draw how the water reacted with the words written in Japanese **"Love/Appreciation"** on the bottle.

Draw how the water reacted with the words written in Japanese **"Dirty"** on the bottle.

Describe the changes you see. Why do you think there are these changes?

How can you apply what Dr. Emoto's research shows into your own life?

Since we are made up of a large percentage of water, how important is it for us to say beautiful and positive words to ourself and others?

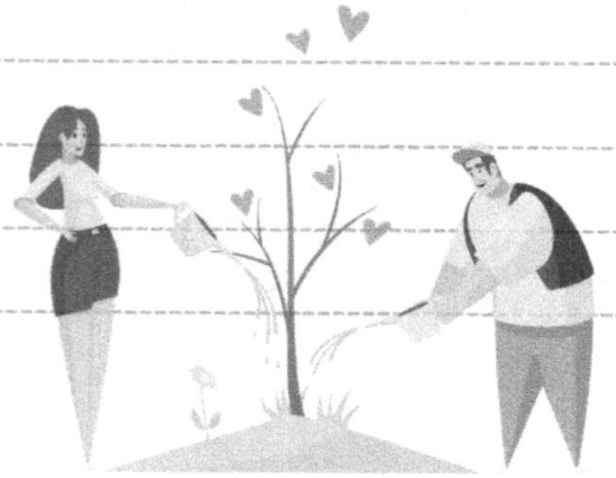

Name some music you think would have a positive effect on water.

Name a few places that would have a positive effect on water.

List a few messages you want your water to "feel" or "resinate."

Under your water, place a note of one message. Try for a week and make note of the effects you experience.

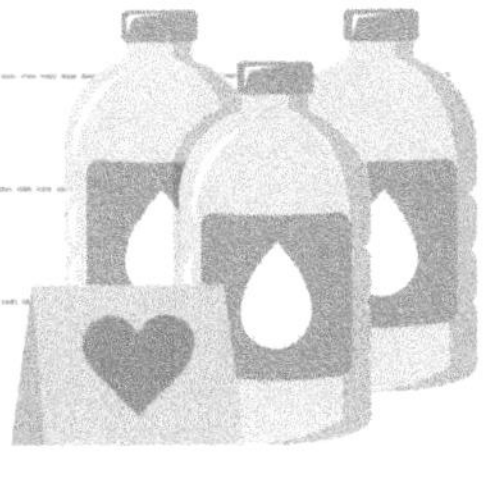

Types of Wet Water

Do you think different filtrations or sources of water would have different results, as in Dr. Emoto's studies? Explain.

Is there an importance to filtering your water? Explain.

List and describe as many different methods to filtering water.

Describe the differences between these types of waters: city tap, well, spring, distilled, rain, aquifer, and bottled. Is one better than the other?

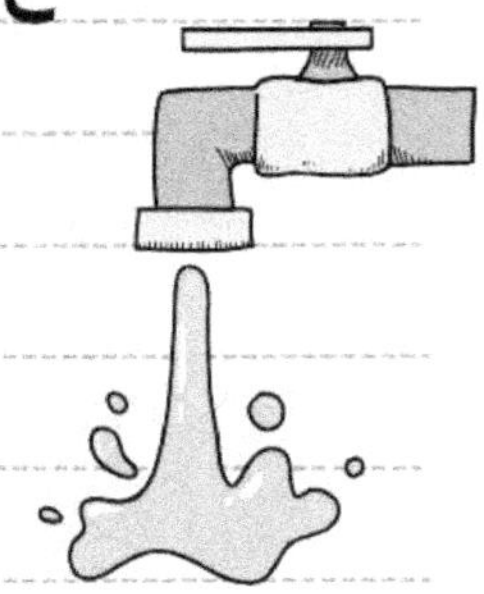

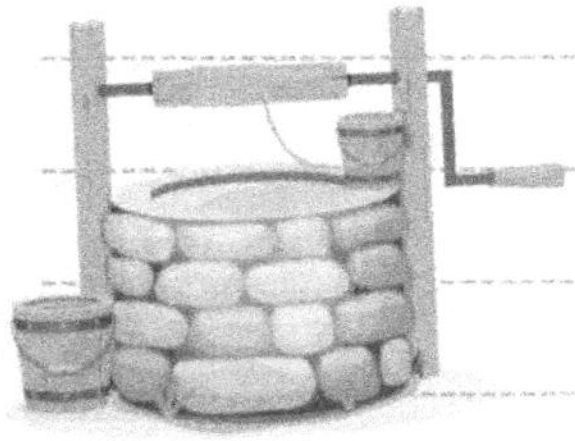

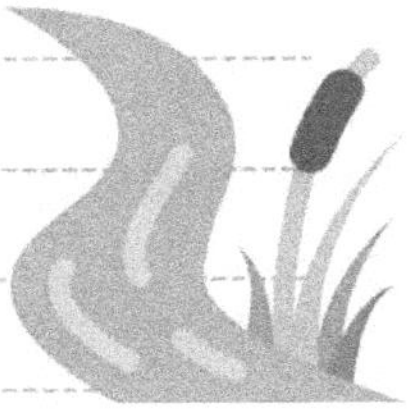

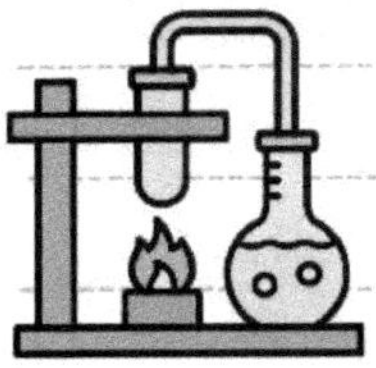

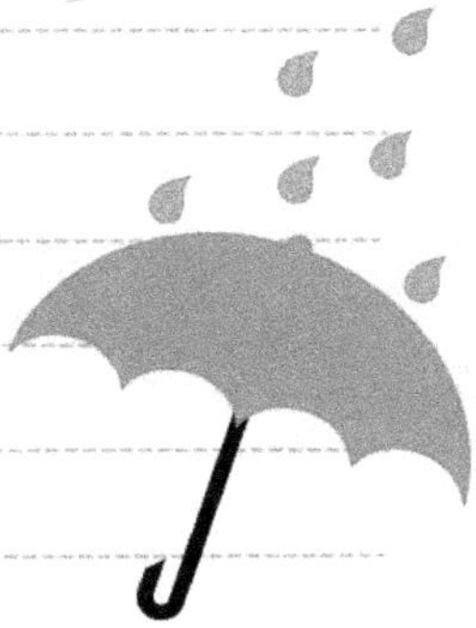

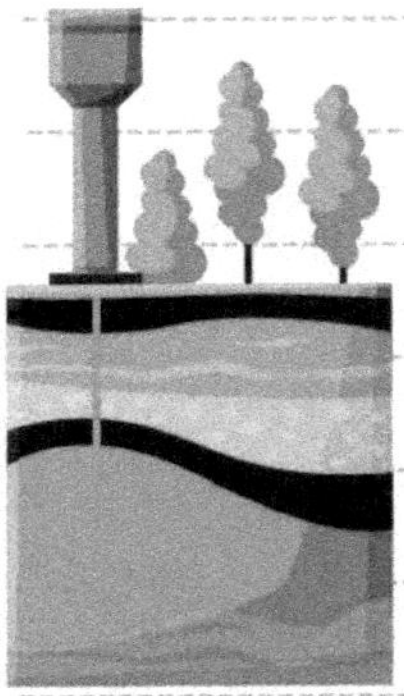

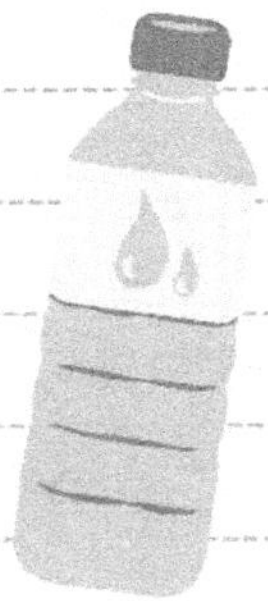

Healthy Juice

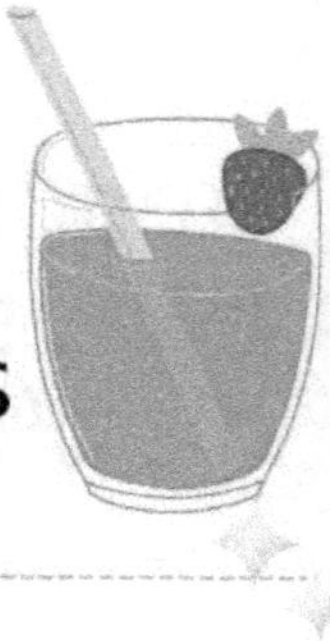

What medicinal and healthy properties make these foods so grand?

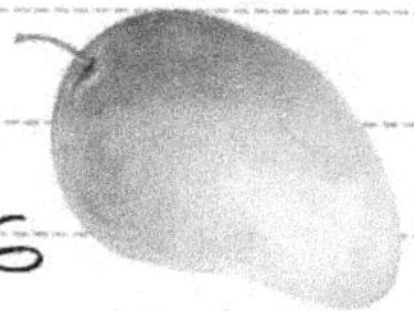

mango

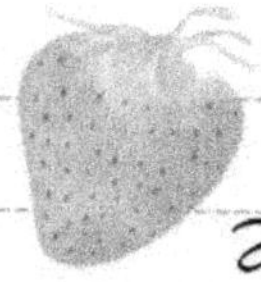

strawberry

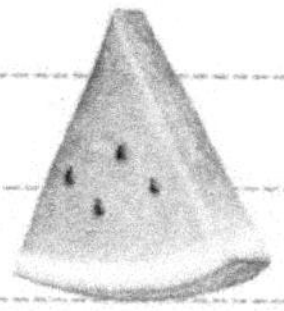

watermelon

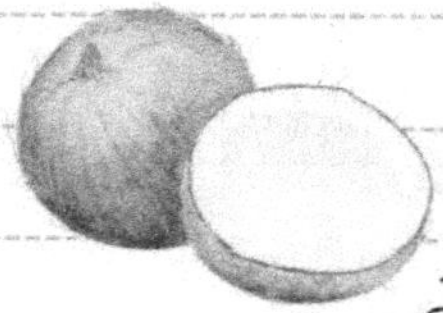

coconut water

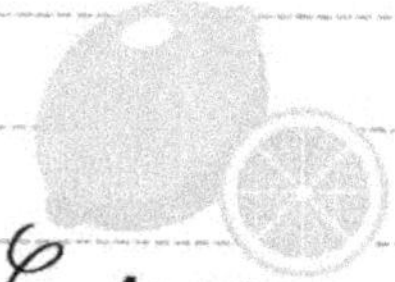

lemon

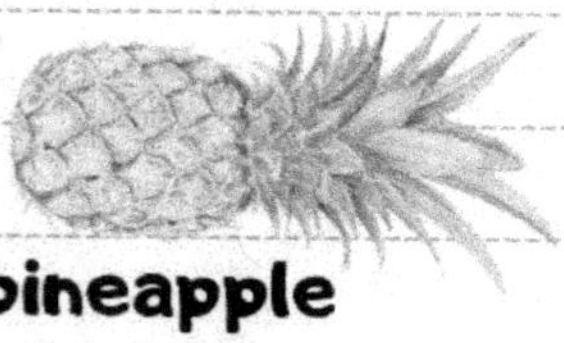

pineapple

Freezing juices in ice cube trays can be an excellent way to make a smoothie refreshingly cold. When freezing your juices, write affirmations or other kind words on a piece of paper and place it under or around your ice cube or popsicle trays. What do you notice?

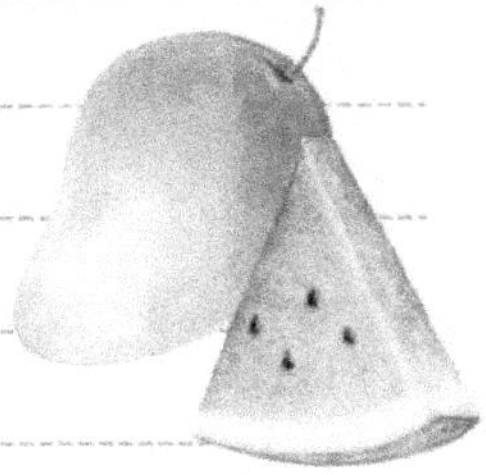

Do some juices freeze better than others? Explain why.

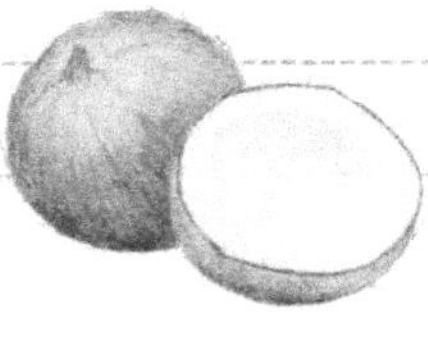

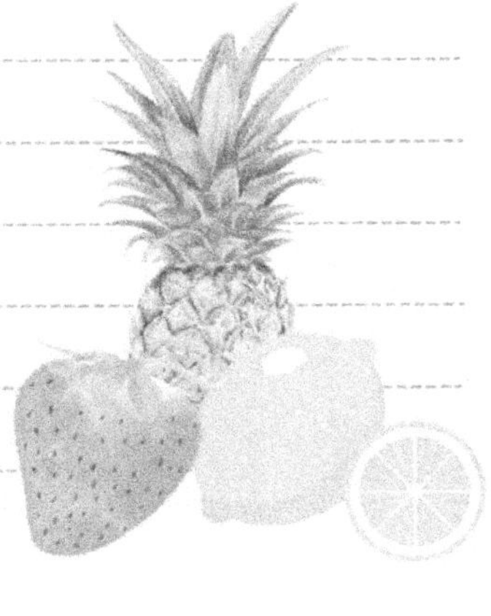

MELON *Slush*

INGREDIENTS

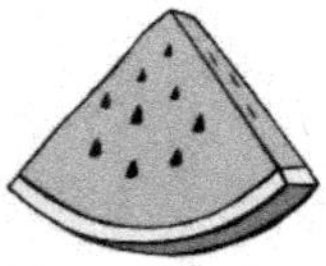

Watermelon

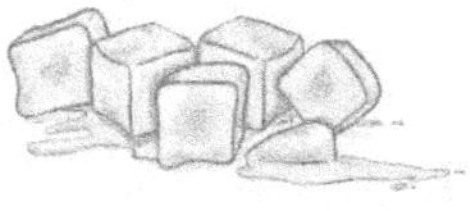

Ice Cubes

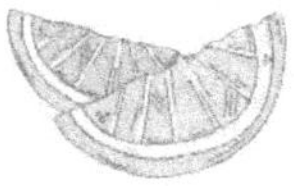

Lemon Juice

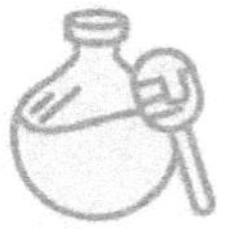

Honey

BLEND TOGETHER & ENJOY

2 cups Watermelon 1/2 cup Ice Cubes	1 Juiced Lemon 1-3 Tablespoons Honey

Slushy Reflection Time

What other liquids could you freeze to substitute the ice cubes, instead of water?

Would you add mint next time?

Would you make any changes to the ingredients?

Did you use any organic ingredients?

What positive affirmations did or will you write under your ice cubes?

Name a few health benefits this drink has.

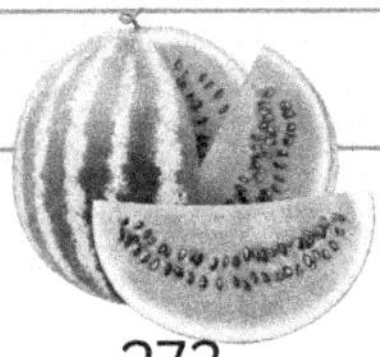

Rewrite your version of the recipe, making changes to quantities, steps, ingredients, or anything else you find fitting.

Recipe Name

Procedure

Yield

Cost

Time

Ingredients

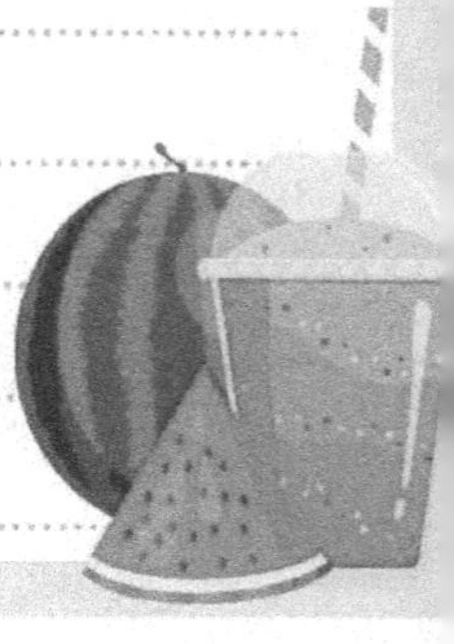

How much would you charge for 16 oz?

What is your profit margin?

Popsicle Freeze

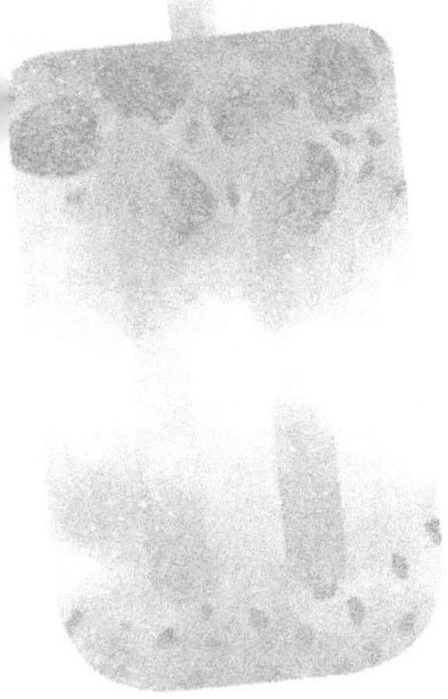

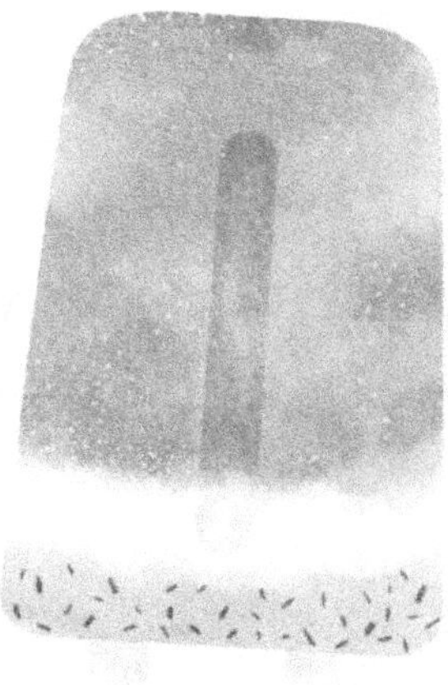

These frozen treats can be a great way to cool off, get a healthy dose of fruits and vegetables, and stay hydrated. Extra bonus: no added sugars needed with the sweetness of fruit!

Research a few recipes, make some, and then try your own. Take notes on supplies and ingredients you will need. Pay attention to the liquid versus solid ratio and the texture. Make adjustments from the ones you tried and customize your own recipe. Take notes along the way.

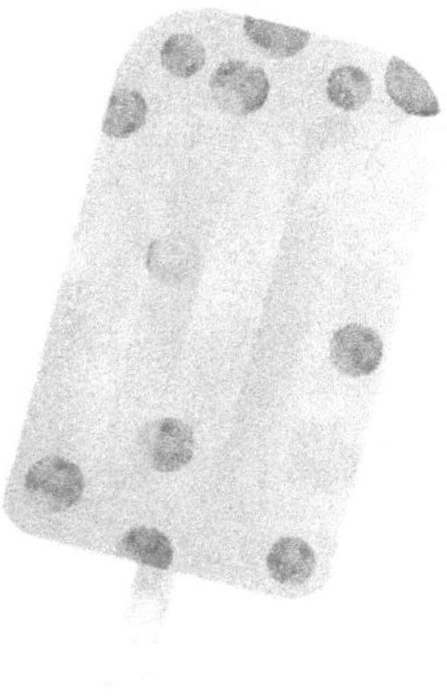

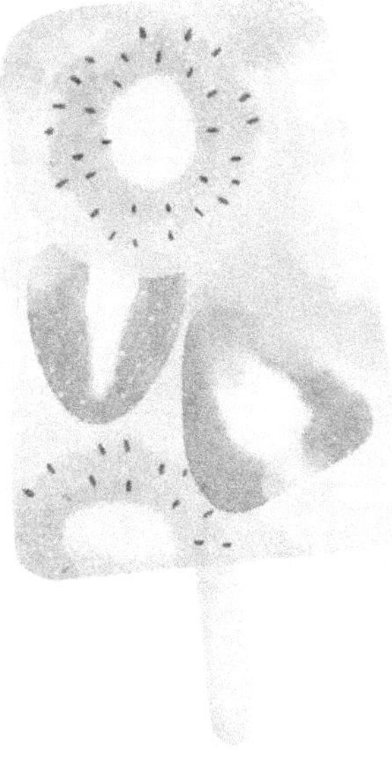

When you make your own recipe, be sure to add your favorite fruits, veggies, liquids, and superfoods.
Have fun and enjoy the journey!

Popsicle Recipe Notes

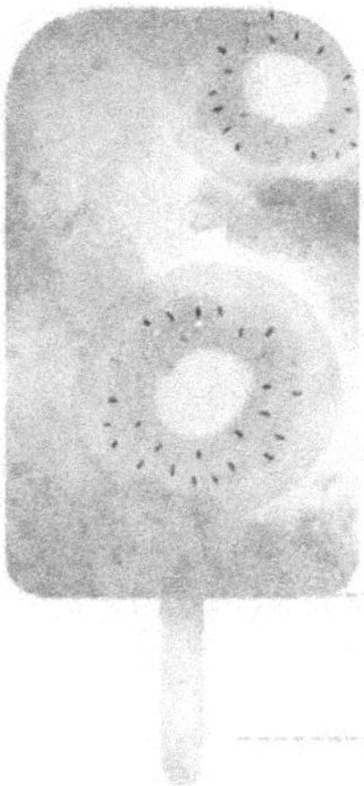

☆☆☆☆☆

Recipe Ingredients:

Liquid to Solid Ratio:

Texture & Taste Description:

Changes/Improvements Needed:

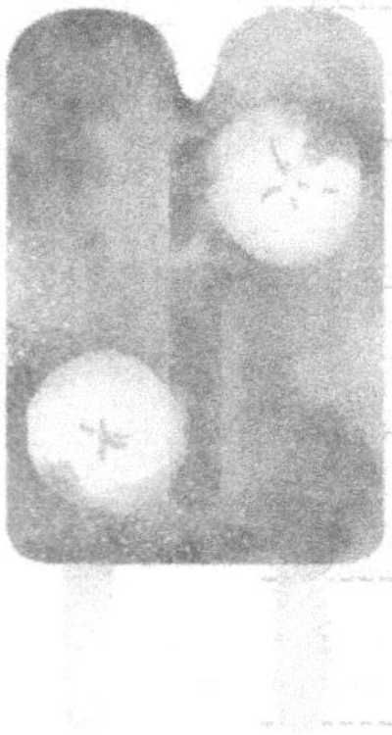

☆☆☆☆☆

Recipe Ingredients:

Liquid to Solid Ratio:

Texture & Taste Description:

Changes/Improvements Needed:

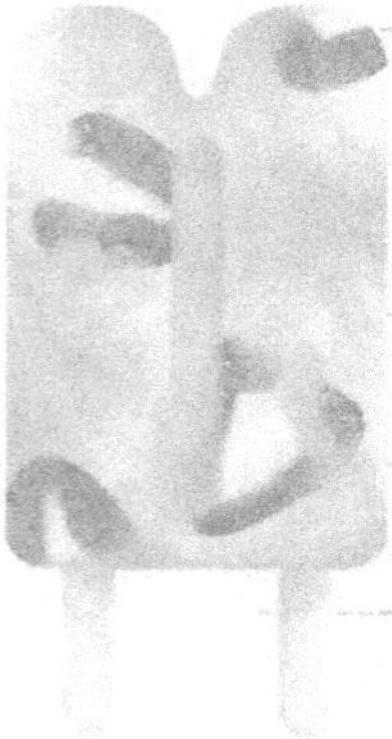

☆☆☆☆☆

Recipe Ingredients:

Liquid to Solid Ratio:

Texture & Taste Description:

Changes/Improvements Needed:

Popsicle Recipe Notes

Recipe Ingredients:

Liquid to Solid Ratio:

Texture & Taste Description:

Changes/Improvements Needed:

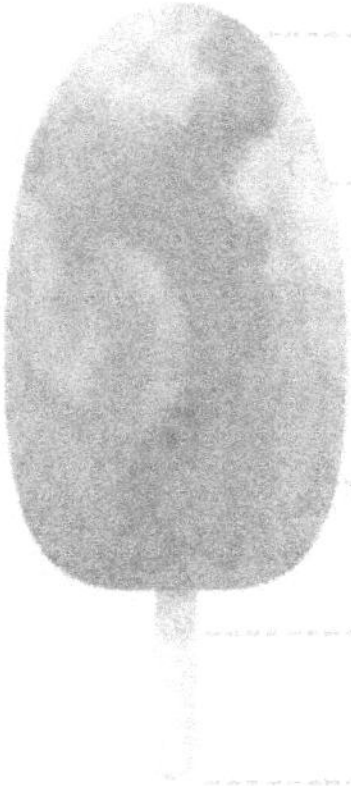

Recipe Ingredients:

Liquid to Solid Ratio:

Texture & Taste Description:

Changes/Improvements Needed:

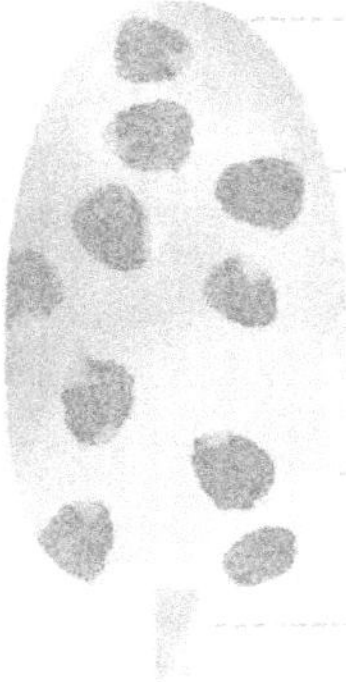

Recipe Ingredients:

Liquid to Solid Ratio:

Texture & Taste Description:

Changes/Improvements Needed:

Write your favorite popsicle recipe.

Recipe Name

Procedure

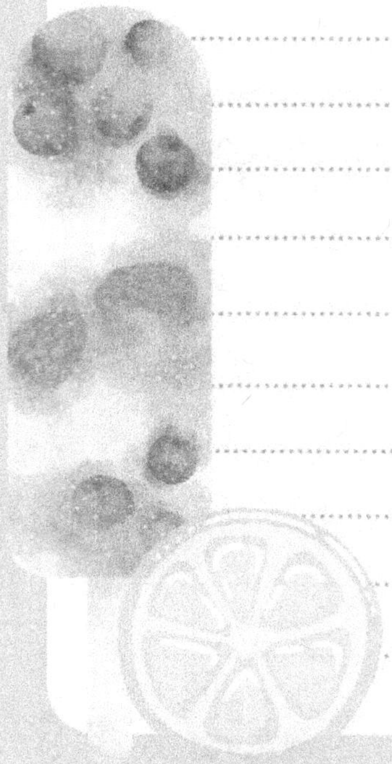

Yield

Cost

Time

Ingredients

How much would you charge for a popsicle?

What is your profit margin?

The Finale

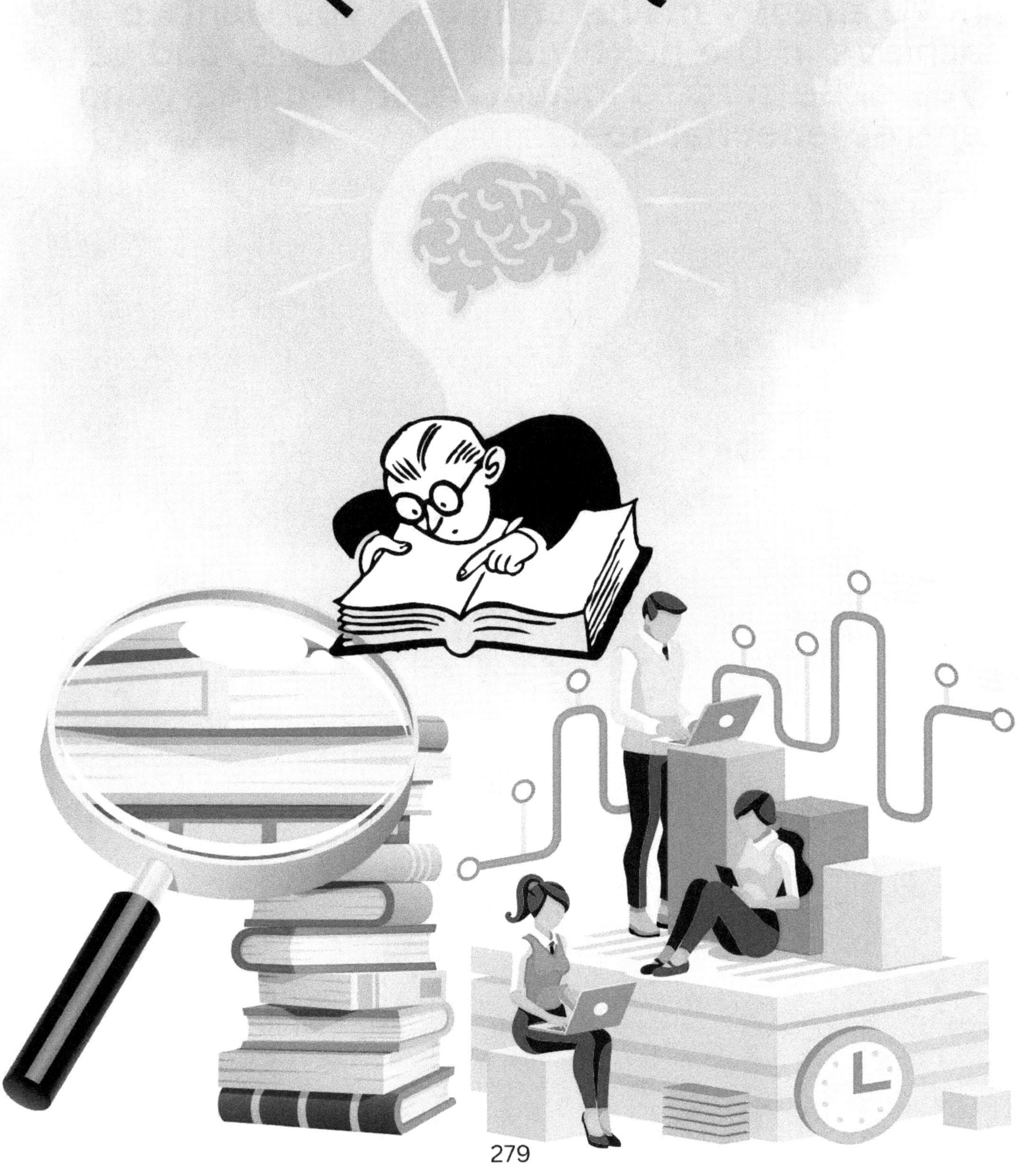

Reflect & Goal Setting

Discuss when you started, the changes you have already made, and what you want to achieve in the next year, five years, and ten years. Be sure to include health, career, and entrepreneurial goals.

Practice your cursive handwriting skills!

Design a nutritional chart, showing each food category. Customize this for you. Include favorite foods that are optimal for your health. For help, reference the food pyramid section at beginning of this book.

Notes:

Go a step further and include healthy habits, such as exercise, meditation, a healthy sleep schedule, breath work, and activities that provide you with internal joy, happiness, and overall fulfillment.

Notes:

Your Nutritional Health Chart:

FOOD TRUCK BUSINESS

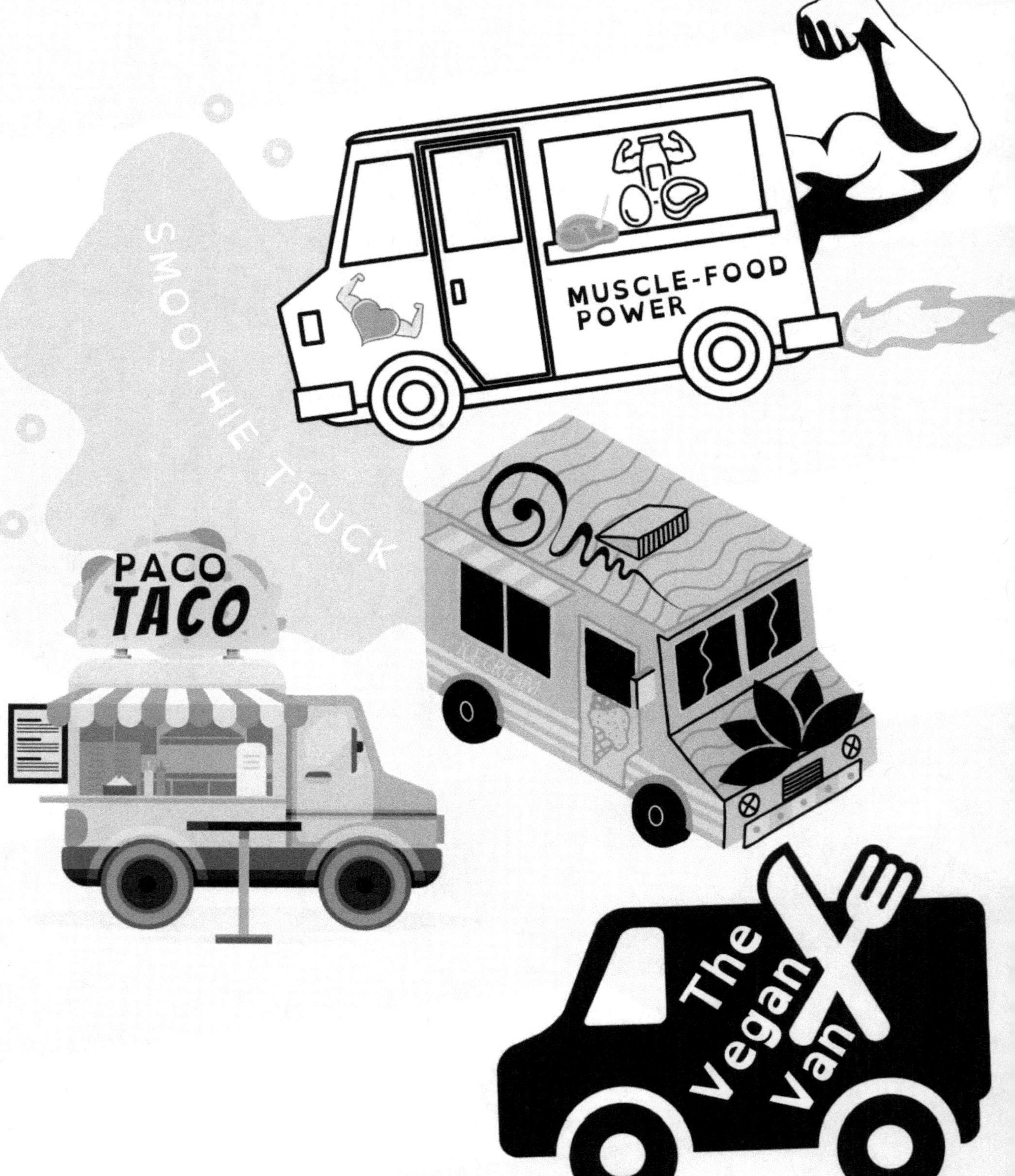

Time to put all your knowledge together from this book, get creative, have fun, and design a food truck business. Your cafe on wheels is to be the healthiest food truck business around. Brainstorm several ideas for the name, theme, slogan or motto for your brand, uniform style for the workers, and anything else that you want for your food truck business.

Draw out your top design ideas.

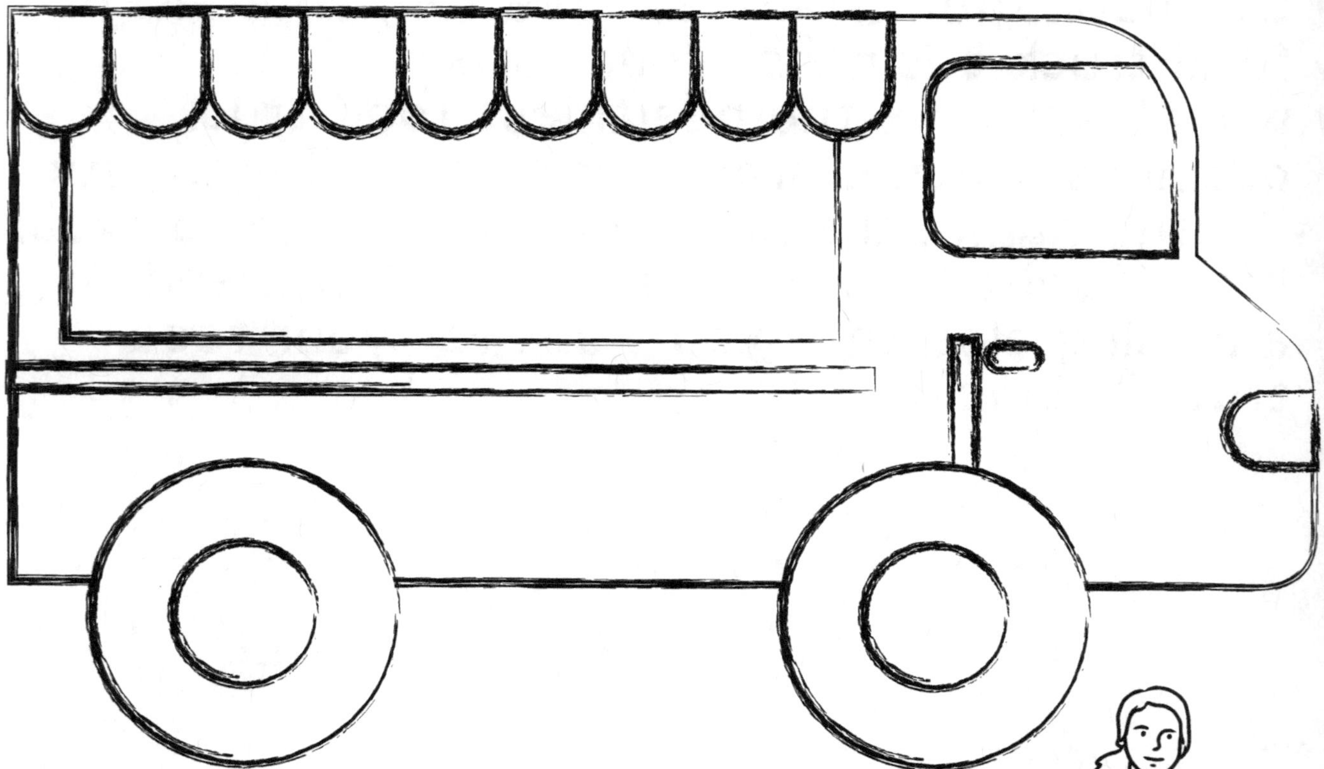

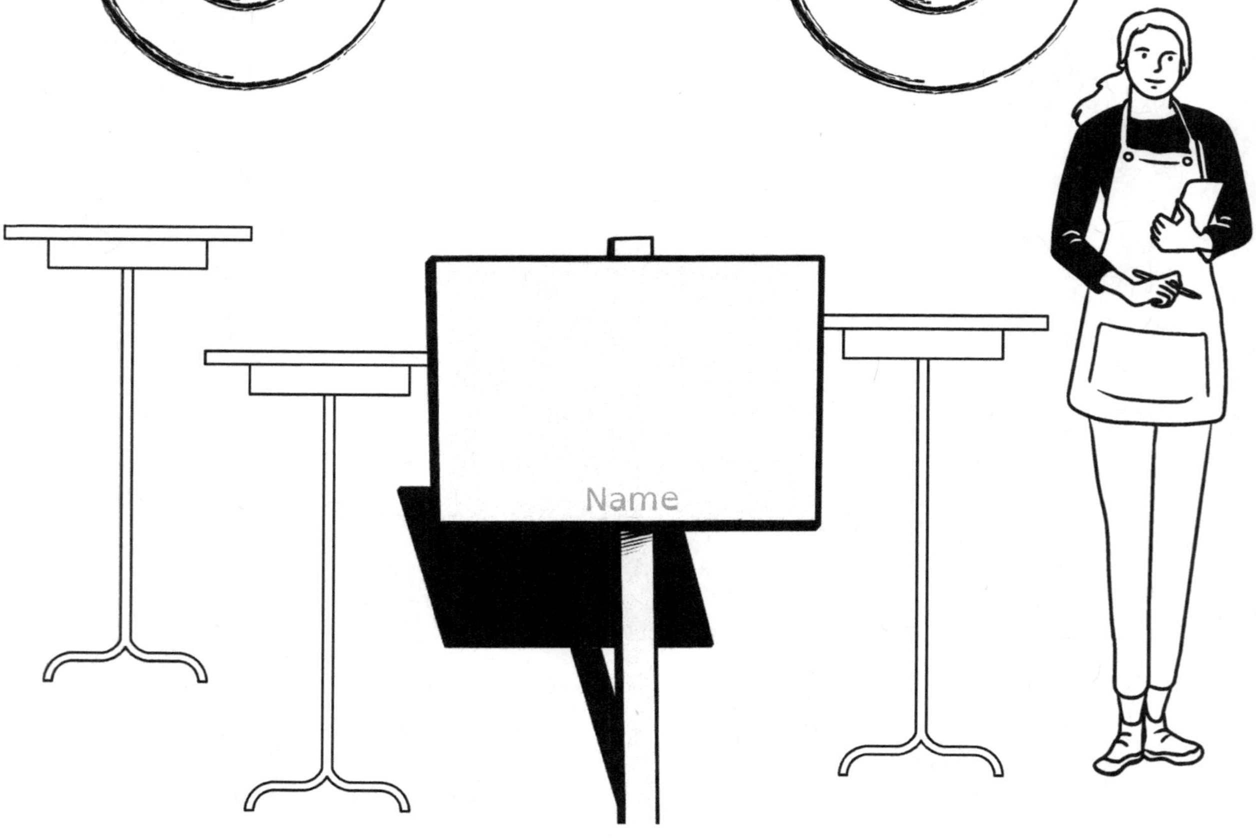

Additional Design Space:

MENU

Use the knowledge you have learned from this book and other sources to create a healthy and balanced menu.

MENU

Can you compare your business to anything that already exists?

What makes your food truck business unique?

What are other ways your truck can promote health of our bodies, minds, and planet?

Food Truck Bonanza

Congratulations, your food truck business has been invited to the world famous Food Truck Bonanza! Time to prepare. Write down everything you will need to pack...food, generators, extension cords, tables, plastic utensils, gasoline/fuel... Research for help.

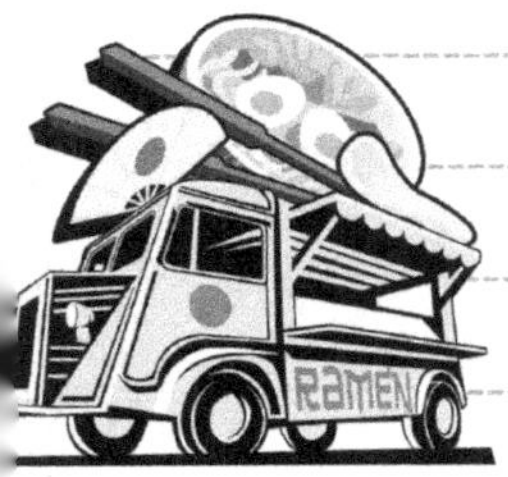

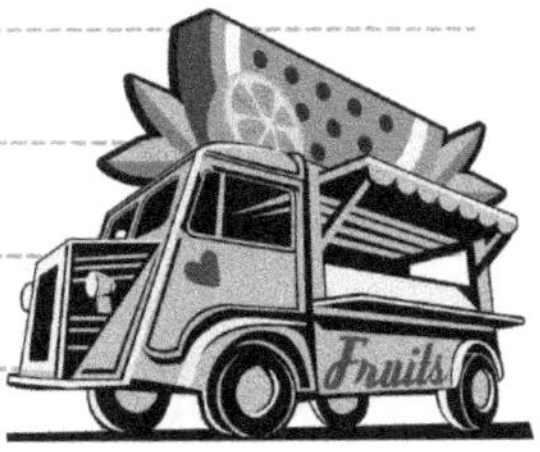

The event is 235 miles away and lasts for 3 days. Your food truck gets 10 miles to the gallon. Gas is $4.27 a gallon. How much will this travel cost to drive there and back?

On average, your trip speed is 40 mph. How long will it take you to travel there and back?

To participate and sell at the Bananza, the fee is $350. How much will the event and fuel cost (expenses) if you commute there and back home each day?

If you decide to stay at a nearby lodging a few miles away for $125 a night, how many nights would you need to stay?

How much would this cost, if you took a one way $12 taxi ride to and from the Bananza each day you stayed at the lodging?

How much time and money would you save by staying in this lodging?

As a business owner, do you decide to stay nearby the Bananza or commute home each night? Explain.

On average, retail foods are priced about 75% more than the cost, to meet profit margins. If a smoothie is on the menu for $10, how much should it cost to make?

How much profit can you make from that smoothie?

How much profit could you potentially make from spending $500 on food to sell?

If you want to profit $1500 during the three day event, how much money would you need to spend on food (food cost)? Remember to adjust for the other expenses first.

Research a couple food truck business, and what their work life is really like. Write down the pros and cons of what you discover.

Would you want to turn this food truck business into reality? Explain.

Dream Stage

Holding onto a dream can be the fuel needed to turn a dream into reality. Step by step, action after action, through struggle and success, then one day, you are living that very dream. Dreaming up a business idea can be the very glue that holds a business together during the difficult times business owners face. Being flexible and having an open mind can help during the growing stages. What skills, habits, or mental techniques help entrepreneurs, business owners, or other successful philanthropists?

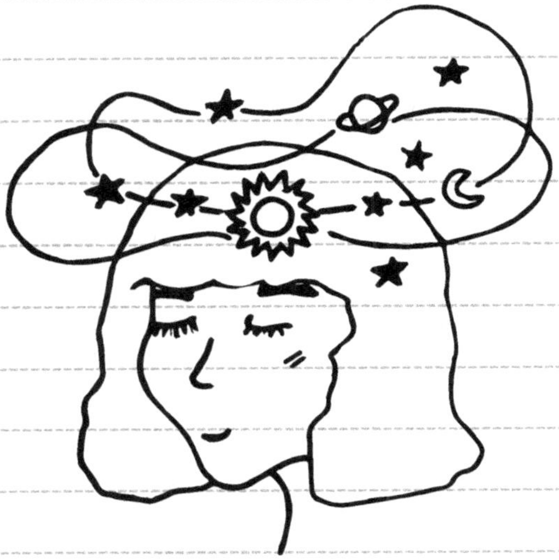

What do you think helps turn a dream into reality? Research this topic in more depth.

Apply these strategies and give examples of what has worked out well.

What other ways can you share a healthy lifestyle with others?

Think creatively about any business ideas that share those same messages as above, write them out.

NOTES, IDEAS, GOALS, AND AFFIRMATIONS

Practice your cursive handwriting skills!

TIME TO CELEBRATE

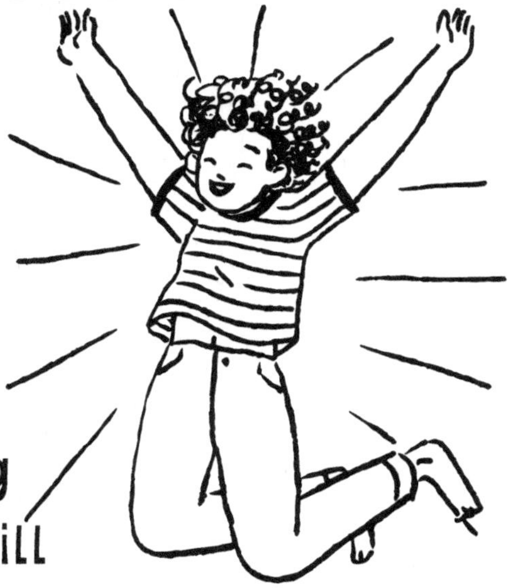

Congratulations!
You did it!
Way to go!

You really have taken a great leap into a beautiful and healthy future. Applying the principles in this book will be a continuous journey in life, ask questions, get excited, have fun, insure your learning and growing never stop. Remember to always seek to invest in yourself: through depositing positive, kind, and loving thoughts and words toward yourself and others, consume nourishing foods that excel your body and mind, and do activities that nourish yourself and inspire the greatness in you!

No one said this would be easy, but would it be worth all the effort? ABSOLUTELY! Believe in yourself, because you are a beautiful being!

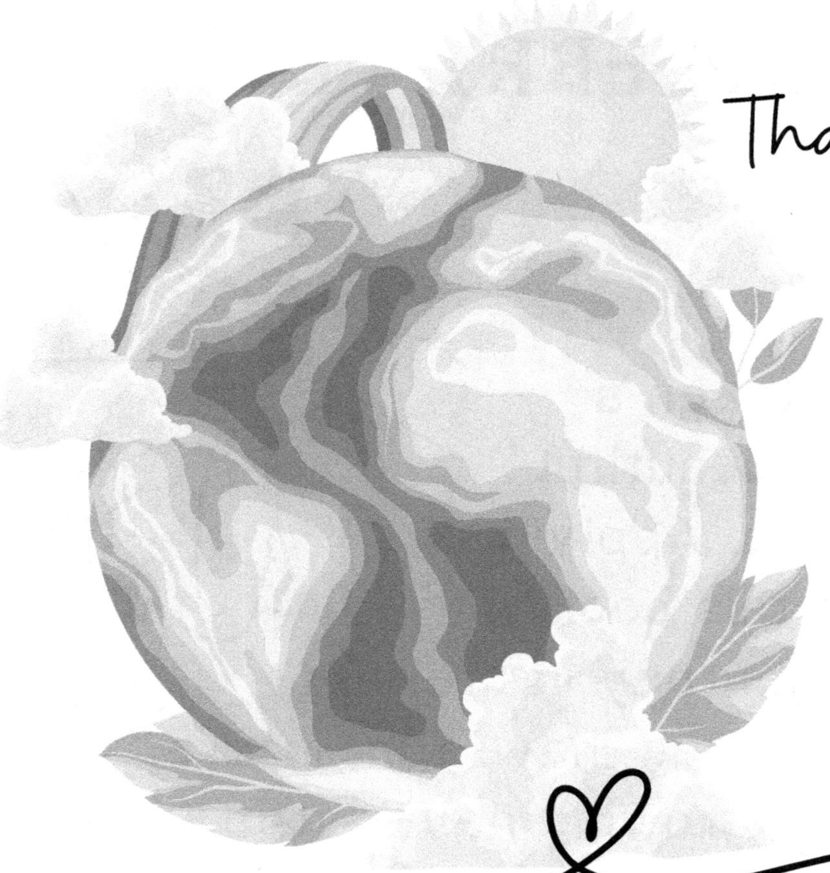

Thank you so much for investing in yourself.

I hope you loved this book!
Please give a review to help others learn about this healthy journey too.

xoxo

Julia Boreck

References

Emoto, M. & I.H.M. *The Message From Water*. General Research Institute. (2000). HADO Kyokusha International. Japan.

EWG. (2022). *BAN CANCER-LINKED CHEMICAL FOUND IN CITRUS!* https://act.ewg.org/UOUNqQZubEqMFeX_xZjwTg2sourceid=1020155&_ga=2.27529268.949922967.1648677816-479892281.1648677816

Fallis. (2021).*The 9 Most Promising Psychobiotics for Anxiety.* https://www.optimallivingdynamics.com/blog/the-9-most-promising-psychobiotics-for-anxiety

Griswold, Maggie. (2020). 11 Filling Superfood Smoothie Recipes To Consoder For Lunch Today. https://stylecaster.com/superfood-smoothie-recipe/

Hernandez, Jen. RDN, CSR, LDN. (2021). PRAL: Understanding Potential Renal AcidLoad For Kidney Disease. https://www.plantpoweredkidneys.com/pral/#PRAL_Alkaline_Foods

NBI. (2022). *How to Use Food as Medicine.https://www.nbihealth.com/how-to-use-food-as-medicine/*

Nunez, Demian & Potter, Madeline. (2020). *Neonicotinoids: the good, the bad, and the ugly.* https://entomology.umd.edu/news/neonicotinoids-the-good-the-bad-and-the-ugly

Sandia, Laura Blu. (2019, Oct. 14). Cacao-Superfood of the Gods. https://medium.com/cacao-ceremonies/cacao-food-of-the-gods-b000297e0537

Stepaniak, J. (2015). The acid-alkaline diet: Balancing the body naturally. Healthy Living Publications.

Zerbe, L., M. S. N. A. S. M.-C. P. T. N. A. S. M.-C. E. S. (2021, March 17). Dirty Dozen List: Are You Eating the Most Pesticide-Laden Produce? Dr. Axe. https://draxe.com/health/dirty-dozen/

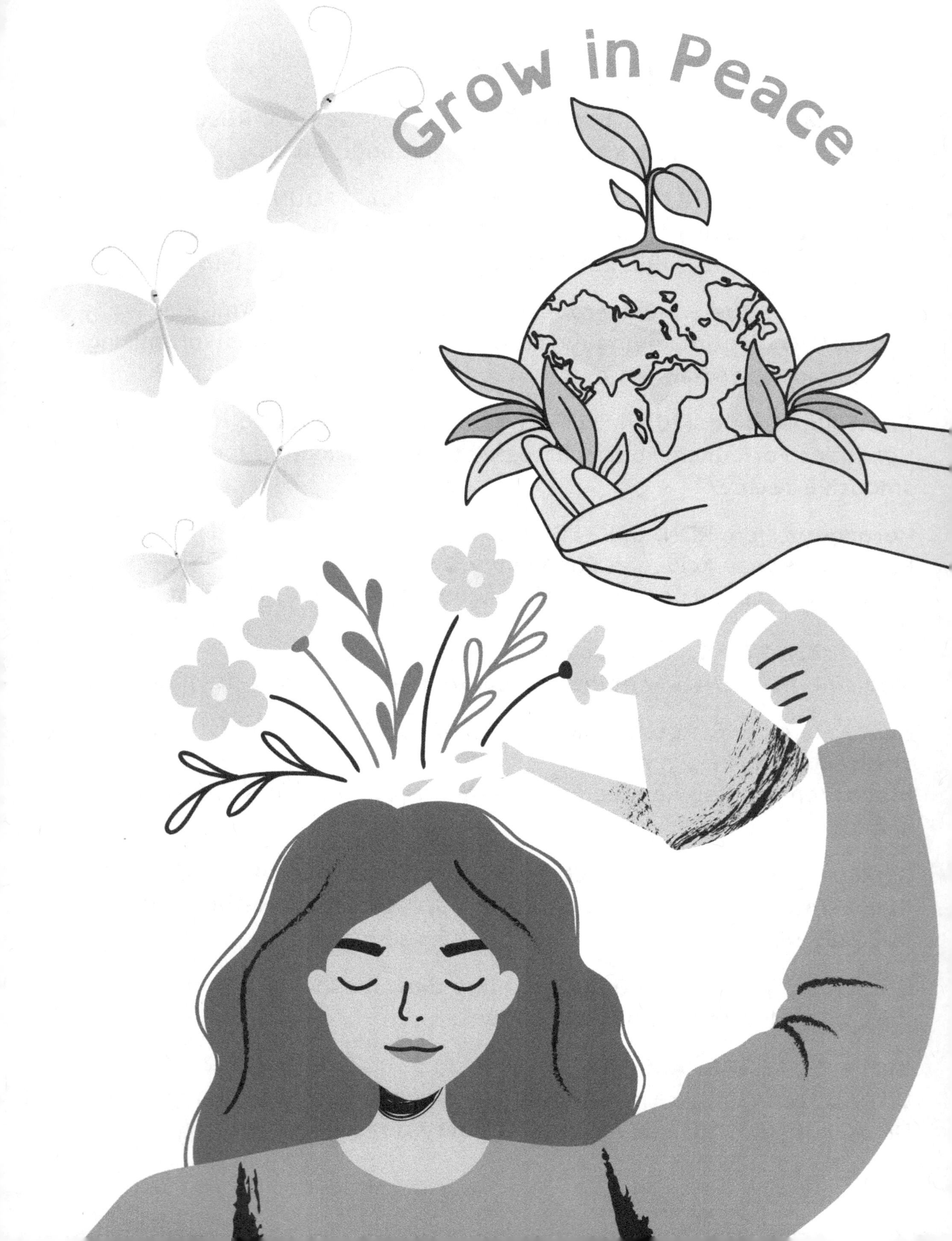
Grow in Peace

www.ingramcontent.com/pod-product-compliance
Lightning Source LLC
LaVergne TN
LVHW060544061126
851857LV00017B/1894
9798988622581